HEALTH AND CULTURE

THEN AND NOW

Collins O. Airhihenbuwa

U-RISE

www.u-rise.org

Dedication

Then:

To my late Parents

My father, Obadolor Airhihenbuwa

My mother, Igbinosa Osomwota

My other father (my wife's father), Jean-Victor Kingue

That we may carry the touch you have passed on to us with the strength, humility, and wholesomeness that you always embodied.

Now:

To all my siblings, past and present, and particularly my brother, Daniel Owa, who joined the ancestors earlier this year, 2025, his humility and nurturing spirit remain an enduring guiderail in my journey.

Contents

Preface

In the introduction to this book, in 1995, I began with a quote by Chinua Achebe: "Where one thing stands, another must stand beside it." He asserted that there is never a single lens through which we are to understand how people from different cultures and contexts make sense of the world. Beyond embracing this notion of multiple truths, *Health and Culture: Beyond the Western Paradigm* was published at a time when International/global health was based on the medical model as well as measures of national development, primarily socioeconomic factors such as education and income. These measures of development were subsequently emphasized in the objectives of the Sustainable Development Goal and its predecessor, the Millennium Development Goal. Thus, development measures and the medical model were the twin global health engines that framed our being in terms of how we were to see deficits in our health status, and thus how we made unhealthy decisions. These framings of global health inevitably focused on implementing health interventions at the individual level. This became the cornerstone of defining and shaping public health, health promotion, and health communication. At the personal level, public health, health promotion, and health communication largely focused on whether individuals accepted or rejected prescribed messages to improve their health. Collective well-being was measured using national development indices derived from Western-based economic productions. Yet, none of these indices considered who we are as cultural beings, or how our decisions, health, and otherwise, are shaped by our cultural, environmental, and political contexts.

As I argued then, culture and identity are always part of our everyday experience, but these experiences tend to be surfaced when our identity and values are in conflict with deployed health messages, and, in that moment, we become the Other. These experiences of being "othered" because one's identity is thought to be irrelevant in health decisions led me to pose the question: *Do you know who you are without what you do?* Today, this self-reflective question that should be the foundation for implementing health interventions in any community is understood as articulating one's positionality. In the past three decades of the publication of the first edition of this book, there have been global events that continue to reveal the falsehood in total reliance on economic development indices for understanding decisions around the prevention of diseases. Indeed, two global events that should have forced us to question our reliance on the lens of disease rather than on the context of health decisions were HIV/AIDS in the 80s and 90s, and COVID-19 today. Each pandemic revealed how our understanding of a global health problem, and our framing of solutions, must value cultural contexts over singular behavior change narratives. The urgency of collective actions grounded in Achebe's multiple truths, not a single truth, was the original motivation for this book and remains so in this revision, particularly given the present political assault on the institutions and profession of public health.

Thirty years ago, many scholars called for teaching politics in public health to better understand how political environments shape the messaging and communication about risk environments (rather than risk factors) that impact health and well-being. Few would argue against the politics of health today, given how politics has devastated public health infrastructure and priorities. Moreover, 'trust and trustworthiness,' considered critical to promoting equity, has become a central issue in public health engagement. Building trust and sustaining trustworthiness within and between communities and institutions to achieve shared public health goals requires commitment, even when outcomes are uncertain. These questions of trust and commitment manifest in the everyday choices we make when we are confronted with political and social challenges.

In response to the political assault on civil and human rights, particularly its devastating impact on public health, a call was issued early in 2025 for a one-day boycott of retail stores to protest assaults on diversity, equity, and inclusion. When I shared this news with a friend, thinking that he would be happy to join, given his professional position in leading DEI initiatives for his organization, he declined to participate, citing his belief that the effort would be unsuccessful. His response caught me off guard, prompting me to reflect on how many of us employ measures of success in the production economy to success in political and social protests designed to challenge the repressive regime of power. It reminded me of Derrick Bell's call to action, as recalled by Chandra Ford during a training we conducted in New York City: We engage not because we know the outcome, but because we are committed to the process, even when the outcome is unknown. To me, unlike my friend, the boycott was not meant to demonstrate a single measurable outcome but instead to affirm our commitment to a process that will require varied strategies over time. These various strategies are echoed in the reflections throughout this edition. Thus, the 'Then' is the original text with modest tweaks, followed by 'Now,' which are the interviews I conducted with kindred cultural scholars and practitioners. I welcome the opportunities to continue these collective conversations that I coined over 30 years ago as '*polylogues*.'

Acknowledgement

THEN:

I pour libation to my ancestors for their spiritual foundations on which the seed of my intellectual curiosity continues to be fertilized and nurtured. My personal and professional growth has been shaped by my Edo cultural values and meanings, on which my humanity is affirmed and legitimized. My humanity continues to be fulfilled by the sense of cultural awareness and pride that was instilled in me by my late mother and father.

A debt of gratitude is owed to many people for their encouragement and support in the completion of this book. First and foremost is my wife, Angele M. Kingue, for the challenge her intellectual, cultural, and moral insights have kindled in me. My son, Iyare, for the inspiration I draw from his perseverance and the sober reminder that the measure of human progress is a matter of how far we have journeyed rather than a marker at some distant point in our destination. My brother, Osa, for his unwavering support in the review of the initial draft of this book. My dear friend Linden Lewis for his painstaking efforts in providing detailed and insightful feedback for a draft of this book. Linden has been particularly generous with his intellectual richness by providing me with important essays and critiques, and his brotherly support in nurturing our kindred spirit. I am thankful to Emmanuel Eze for his critique and feedback in the preparation of this book. I owe a debt of gratitude to my friend and mentor, James B. Stewart, for his towering and unequivocal support over the years. Jim has been a guiding light in providing feedback on the preparation of several of my published articles. This book was no exception. His thorough and selfless dedication to excellence has become a model to which I aspire.

Many thanks go to several of my students over the years, from whom I have learned so much. There are too many to identify by name, and yet I feel obliged to name two of them. Leonard Jack,

Jr, with whom I have collaborated on several projects and who continues to be a close and valued friend and colleague; and Michael Ludwig, who has deepened my appreciation for dialogical education in more than one way. In preparing this book, I drew on the many writings of outstanding educational theorists and cultural critics. Among them is Henry Giroux, whom, through personal interaction, I have been fortunate to have gained an unparalleled intellectual stimulation. He has been very generous with his time in providing me with valuable feedback on a draft of this book.

So many others have directly and indirectly nourished my scholarly appetite as well as enriched my personal and professional growth. They include, Shiriki Kumanyika, Dory Storms, Richard Smith, and Cathy Lyons. I am grateful to my co-authors, Ira Harrison and Agatha Lowe, Ralp DiClemente, and Gina Wingood, with whom I published the original version of two of the chapters in this book. Finally, I would like to thank Sage Publications editors Christine Smedley, Diane Foster, and Judy Selhorst for their support in the book production.

While the support for me has been extensive across my personal and professional extended family, all mistakes and errors in this book are solely mine.

NOW:

I continue to pour libation to my ancestors, whose spiritual foundations nurture the seed of my personal and intellectual curiosity, allowing it to take root, grow, and flourish. I remain most humbled by the love and support I continue to receive from family and kindreds. My son, Yannick, was born after the first edition of this book, and his growth, maturity, and caring personality bring me joy each day as I see my own childhood and young adult years through his strong sense of purposeful selfhood. To Angele, my wife, for her love, encouragement, and decades of mutually inspiring conversations grounded in our shared and unwavering commitment to re-imagining language in ways that give depth and breadth to African ways of knowing. As part of launching the original book in 1995, I remain deeply grateful to Kathleen Roe, the first academic leader who invited me to discuss the book with her San José State University Public Health students, and to Bunmi Makinwa, who invited me to engage his health, communication, and international development colleagues in Nairobi, Kenya. When it comes to the decision to embark on this edition, no one deserves more credit than Juliet Iwelunmor, whose steady encouragement and nudges over the past year pushed me to bring it to completion. I have benefitted immensely from our numerous collaborations over the years, as well as our shared love for creating spaces for radical cultural healing. Following the successful webinar she and her WashU LIGHT Center team hosted to mark the 30th anniversary of *Health and Culture*, it became clear that this edition was not only timely but necessary. I have benefited greatly from the scholarly vision and commitments of the contributors in the NOW of this edition, especially the contributors with whom I have had the privilege of co-producing knowledge as students, who have now emerged as public health frontline leaders, activist scholars/practitioners, and cultural path breakers. To that end, I remain ever grateful to every contributor to the reflection in each chapter of this edition. Each person, from those with over 40 years of experience and commitment to this work to those at the early stage of their journey, remains a champion in valuing culture, beyond the Western Paradigm. Your willingness to be part of this new edition is a testament to your commitment to health and culture globally. In completing the production process of this book,

I am grateful to Shaina Amienyi for her support, professionalism, and patience in preparing the initial layout, and to Bianca Kipp for bringing into production the book cover I had generated. Many of my kindred scholars have supported my work over the years and remain allies in this journey. In particular, I am grateful to Teri Murray for always sharing her rich professional insights as she did in her thorough review and thoughtful editorial comments on a draft of these conversations. In the NOW sections of this edition, I note that AI was used to improve clarity, flow, and conciseness while maintaining the original conversation ideas and meanings. Finally, I am grateful to Leyla Carter and the BookBaby Publishing editorial team, for copyediting, layout, and final production work.

As I stated in the original publication, while the support for me has been extensive across my personal and professional extended family, all mistakes and errors in this edition are solely mine.

Introduction

THEN:

> Where one thing stands, another thing must stand beside it...This saying "there is only one way" is something which is new to my people.
>
> Chinua Achebe

The African philosophy of life, invoked by Achebe in the above epithet, is the bedrock on which the discourse in this book is grounded. This philosophy of human construction of reality, as lived in many African cultures, underscores an embracing of multiple truths relative to health, education, politics, religion, valuation, and thus decision-making processes. This ideology, which shuns the "All or nothing" mentality of Western culture and its attendant promotion of universal truths, should be understood not only for its counterpoising principle and quality but as a different genre.

This book challenges traditional paradigms in health, education, and development on three primary, yet complementary fronts. The first is the valorizing of Eurocentrism and Patriarchy in the production and acquisition of health knowledge and health behavior, while continuing to oppress and suppress cultural expressions of non-Western peoples and women. The second principle is the reliance on the notion of "development" as an emancipatory process, even though this concept is grounded in the promotion of Western hegemony in the name of universal progress. Development ideology valorizes standardization through the notion of universal truths in the name of a common global mission. The third principle, which directly relates to the first two, is the overemphasis of health promotion and disease prevention practices on the medical model of prevention. Consequently, the fields of public health and health education/promotion have failed to ground their professional (both philosophical and practical) praxis adequately in such areas of the humanities as philosophy, language, history, cultural and critical studies. The result has been the absence of meaningful participation of people and their culture in advancing positive health behavioral transformation where appropriate. It has become a common practice in public health, social, and behavioral sciences to vocalize the importance of culture in studying and understanding health behaviors, even though culture is yet to be inscribed at the primacy of public health promotion and disease prevention programs, at least not in any manner that legitimates its centrality in public health praxis.

Public health and Health promotion practices continue to operate under the strong and direct influence of the Westernized medical model of prevention. While certain benefits are derived from such influence, it seems unconscionable that a profession that anchors its *raison d'etre* on the ability to influence human behavior has consistently undermined and, in most cases, ignored the centrality of culture (as evident in the mission of critical cultural studies, for example) in health, communication, and education. There continues to be a strong public health reliance on clinical medicine and individual psychology, even though these lenses for public health have constantly been challenged for their limitations, which are driven by monocentrism, resulting in cultural erasures. For example, Chow (1991) concluded that psychoanalysis is a Western practice that focuses on the private self, whereas the Chinese and many other non-Western cultures are more concerned with public life and the larger issues of history rather than privacy. Thus, psychoanalysis as a function of the private self is culturally disconnected from the notion of collective identity evident in many non-Western countries. Public health, therefore, must learn from the limitations in approaches used by Western `development' specialists in their attempt to focus only on individual behavior to guide societal change in non-Western nations.

The ideology behind the concept of development has reified Western hegemony by anchoring measures of "progress" on the values and principles of the West. "Only from the vantage point of the West is it possible to define the 'third world' as underdeveloped and economically dependent. Without the overdetermined discourse that creates the third world, there would be no (singular and privileged) first world" (Mohanty, 1991, P 74). Development conceived of as a prepackaged formula that is only manufactured in Northern nations for application in Southern nations is now an outmoded construct (Sachs, 1992). This concept, with its appropriation of Southern nations as "underdeveloped," was injected into popular discourse on January 20, 1949, by Harry S. Truman. After more than forty years (*now more than 70 years and counting*) of exposing the historical genealogy of the disempowering and non-participatory nature of the concept of development, a new concept is invoked that is equally disempowering since it promises to further marginalize the cultural expressions of Southern nations--Globalization. Although globalization, as theorized from a political, sociological, economic, environmental, geographic, and even historical perspectives, may not have been intended to become a signifier of "progress" but rather a process of integration and incorporation of national economies into a global one, its appropriation in the areas of health and human development as "a marker for progress" has become the inevitable outcome.

Globalization has now been introduced into popular discourse at the *fin de siecle* as the new language of universal truth. The life support of globalization rests on fulfilling the 'needs' of the "Wretched of the Earth" and the "Faces at the Bottom of the Well". "Just as 'needs' became an important emblem which allowed managers to provide a philanthropic rationale for the destruction of cultures, so, now, needs are being replaced by the new emblem of 'basic requirements' under which the new goal, 'survival of the earth' can be justified" (Illich, 1992, p. 98). Like its predecessor, development, globalization is *acultural* and promises to further medicalize and psychologize, in the western sense, human behavior such that non-western cultures are expected to maintain their "underdeveloped" state and play catch-up, as it is currently the case in many African and global south countries.

The present investigation is undertaken with the premise that African theory and practice, particularly within the context of health, must be based on African cultural codes and meaning. The focus here is not on cultural relativism but rather on problematizing the notion of universal truth. In explicating African cultural productions, "Western interpreters as well as African analysts have been using categories and conceptual systems which depend on a Western epistemological order." (Mudimbe, 1988, p.x). This is particularly salient in the discourse of health and education in Africa. Progressive discourses/theories of today - postmodern, postcolonial, feminist, and cultural studies - have challenged classical paradigms by advocating for representation or what Stuart Hall calls the "third space". However, these theories/discourses have failed to adequately address health as a cultural production. While the various inputs into cultural production are shaped by elements of the fields of humanity, the output of cultural production is realized in the health status of individuals and the health conditions of societies.

To invoke the centrality of culture in public health and public health activities is to challenge health promotion and disease prevention approaches that overlook or downplay the importance of history, politics, and education in shaping the landscape of cultural production. Further, it is also to deepen and extend the possibilities of progressive approaches, as in critical pedagogy and critical cultural studies, that centralize culture in its theory and practice. To accomplish these tasks, the deconstruction of existing systems of dominant values must be done in a manner that challenges the very foundation of the social and cultural order. Such a challenge is not merely to destroy a few prejudices; rather, it is to see through the revolving door of all rationalizations by meeting head-on the truth of the struggle between fictions and reality (Minh-Ha, 1991). The centrality of culture in public health, communication, and education initiatives is a discourse that resonates with the politics of representation, which are affirmed through voices of various cultural expressions and meanings. Cultural workers who are engaged in the politics of representation seek to deconstruct (analyzing the historical genealogy) the anthropologization of meaning that has become normative in many health promotion and disease prevention programs. Stated differently, the terrain of public health interventions and programs is replete with appropriation of pejorative cultural codes and meanings that are anchored in Eurocentric and westernized ideology. The tension that results from this misappropriation is manifested in the practices of behavioral and social scientists, such as anthropologists, (even with the best of intentions), whose actions, by the nature of their professional episteme, imply the silence of "Others". An unresolvable problem of anthropology is essentially that it is a discourse of representation of "Others" who are defined epistemologically as inferior, silent, and should be spoken for (Said, 1990). In the words of Trinh T. Minh-Ha (as quoted by Linda Alcoff), anthropology is "mainly a conversation of `us' with `us' about `them', of the white man with the white man about the primitive-nature man... in which `them' is silent." p.6.

In the United States, the appropriation of Jazz by external interests and translation into symbolic representations that allow mimicry is an example of how anthropologizing is operationalized within a culture and can manipulate the cultural rules in ways not conceivable by those who birth and nurture such a cultural production (Stewart, 1992). Although the concern about speaking for others has always been focused on anthropologists, the fact remains that many behavioral and social scientists, including the Public Health, Health Promotion, and communication professionals, engage in anthropologization of meaning. In their desire to raise the level of awareness about non-Western cultures, these professionals ground their theory and practice in a Westernized gaze. By so doing, they often obscure and distort the meaning of what they observe, and thus the reporting and messaging of what has been observed. When this occurs, even though it may be inadvertent, the outcome is misrepresentation of cultural codes and meaning of the non-Western cultures. Such misappropriation dehistoricizes cultural values and meaning while truncating their cultural genealogy and transformative strength and possibilities. What often results is the periodization of cultural practices as archival remains, invoking a notion that the present has no link to the past and thus erasing any historical continuity. Yet, the most efficient cultural weapon with which a people can arm itself is the feeling of historical continuity (Diop, 1981).

Cultures and traditions are simply the forms of social interaction accepted by a particular community at a particular time, and according to its world-view and historical experiences, such that there are several alternatives and systems of values that are selected for their usefulness (Akinjogbin, 1990). In other words, contrary to popular notions, culture is NOT past values and practices that have fossilized at a particular point in history without ever changing and are only recounted orally in the present. Values and practices that remain in the past and are no longer practiced should not be considered (for all practical purposes) a part of an active culture and tradition. The notion that culture and tradition are those practices that were engaged in the past and therefore should be forgotten only promotes cultural amnesia or worse, cultural erasure. According to Chinweizu (1987), those who would teach us amnesia about our past, especially while doping us with accounts of the past of other people, cannot have our best interests at heart. They wish us to commit social and cultural suicide by turning into zombies.

Cultures are not static. They change over time in accordance with the interpretive values of the beliefs, norms, and practices of the group, whose members define and live by the ideals of those practices and values. Very often, culture is blamed for certain ill-understood health practices, when in fact the culprit is the lofty interpretation of culture for the maintenance of imperial dominance and hegemony. This has been particularly true when Westernized professionals address issues of health beliefs and practices in African societies.

Preventive health programs that are anchored in culturally appropriate paradigms enhance and magnify the possibilities that are offered in progressive educational processes/approaches that embrace a dialogical participation. This process of engaging the teacher/interventionists and the students/audiences in the production of meaning, value, pleasure, and knowledge should be central to the mission of health promotion and education. It is only through such dialogue that varied cultural expressions and meanings are affirmed and centralized, and the production of cultural identity can be legitimizing and empowering relative to promoting individual, family, community, and societal health.

This book has a total of eight chapters. In chapter 1, a discussion of health promotion and the discourse on culture and development is offered. Chapter two magnifies the salience of the theme presented in chapter 1 by focusing on the importance of cultural codes in health communication. Chapter 3 is an introduction to a cultural model (PEN-3) for decolonizing health communication and education programs. This chapter offers an opportunity to link theory with practice in developing health promotion and disease prevention programs. This programmatic method offers the opportunity to understand and evaluate culture from multiple dimensions that include positive aspects of culture instead of appropriating culture only as a barrier. In chapter 4, the historical and cultural context of traditional medicine is presented with examples of how this modality can be strengthened from within its cultural space in order to maximize its benefit for global health. In chapter 5, women's health issues are discussed as a construct of patriarchal hegemony on the one hand and westernized female hegemony on the other. The degree to which these combined forces negate the voices of African women and thus compromise their health status and health concerns, such as menopause, is discussed. Chapter 6 addresses the health concerns of children and youth. The socio-cultural production of youth within the African context is discussed. Health conditions of children and youth are presented to underscore the way in which the silencing of youth by adults has contributed to the condition of poor health and perfidy among youth. Chapter 7 addresses the health concerns of African Americans within the context of culture. Identity formation relative to politics of representation is presented as a backdrop for discussing the way in which culture mediates and is mediated by individual, family, and society. Thus, the challenge of individual possibilities against the weight of societal constraint is discussed within the context of empowerment. The mythology of health care as "a delivery system" is problematized by focusing on the way in which the system renders selective services that are dictated through the power of medical production. In chapter 8, a futuristic approach to health promotion is presented as a challenge to moving beyond the decolonization of health and education as a cultural, political, and educational project. Such a challenge requires that health and education draw from the theory and practice of critical cultural studies and other areas of the humanities rather than placing undue reliance on the medical model to address health problems in Africa.

While the totalizing of African experiences is not always an accurate reflection of its intra-regional diversity, it is often invoked mostly due to the shared colonial and post-colonial experiences and political and economic oppression, which continues to be reinscribed in the policies of international agencies such as the International Monetary Fund, the World Bank, and the World Health Organization. This book invites an opportunity for scholars and cultural workers committed to the politics of representation in public health, communication, education, and development to engage in a `polylogue' designed to create a space in which voices of various intellectual and programmatic discourses are affirmed and legitimized. It recognizes and inscribes culture at the core of understanding and influencing health behavior in a manner that centers the oppressed and marginalized in creating and managing their collective destinies. Such a transformative process reinforces Chinua Achebe's words of wisdom, which have been echoed by Chinweizu, reminding us that the West has not put the final touches to creation because it is morning yet on creation day.

NOW:

On April 7, 2025, a webinar was hosted by Professor Juliet Iwelunmor and her LIGHT Center team at Washington University in St. Louis to mark the 30th anniversary of *Health and Culture,* which was published on April 7, 1995. During the event, I announced the preparation and publication of this new edition, explaining that it would present the original text as "Then" and transcripts of conversational interviews with scholars and practitioners reflecting on each chapter as "Now."

So much has happened in the three decades since 1995. Of the questions posed to me by many scholars and practitioners as I reflect on the book, two questions stood out, and they are: 1) What has changed, and what remains to be done? 2) In what ways do language and storytelling remain central to the future of work in culture and health? Addressing these questions was central to how I framed the interview reflection questions I posed to my colleagues/interviewees, asking them to reflect on the lessons of the past and where those lessons have and should take us. Over the past 30 years, for example, more programs and disciplines have embraced the importance of focusing on the strengths of communities, cultures, and populations, rather than only on deficits. Where the word "barrier" once dominated discussions of culture, "cultural strength" has emerged as a new way to understand ourselves, otherized groups, and what matters to us.

While I do not claim credit for this shift, I note that a subspecialty of positive psychology was established in 1998, just three years after the publication of this book. As knowledge production lenses shifted toward the positive, there was also greater emphasis on addressing the systems and structures that shape and regulate behavior, rather than simply blaming individuals for "poor" behavior.

Despite this progress, the future still calls for resisting the temptation to view culture through a single lens. Instead, we must see culture through multiple lenses that encompass personhood, relationships, and structural environments, which I have framed in the PEN-3 Model as the Person, Extended Family, and Neighborhood. A detailed discussion of how scholars and practitioners have applied

PEN-3 can be found in the book I co-edited with Juliet Iwelunmor, entitled *Health, Culture and Place: From the Tree to the Forest (2022)*. Beyond the model, this book takes us on a cultural journey to advance our understanding of culture's role in health systems, infrastructures, and, ultimately, in creating spaces we can call healthy homes.

As I reflect on my hopes for this 2025 edition, given culture's continued centrality to health, I offer my thoughts on three cross-cutting themes on cultural narratives that were surfaced by my colleagues during the interview - language, storytelling, and hope, all of which remain at the core of how we teach and learn.

Language: On the question of language, I return to my beginnings, growing up as a young Nigerian in an Edo village, raised by parents who were neither lettered, schooled, nor credentialed, yet deeply educated. I was rooted and nurtured in their cultural wealth of wisdom. I was always soaked in Edo cultural waters, surrounded by immense cultural wealth, even if I did not fully appreciate or know how to acknowledge it at the time.

When I came to the United States, I enrolled as an undergraduate at Tennessee State University, a Historically Black College/University (HBCU), where some of my cultural values were reinforced. But it wasn't until I began my graduate training that I encountered the deficit language often used to describe populations experiencing ill health, particularly in African countries. For example, my parents and others in my cultural circle who embodied their values were described as "ignorant," people who needed to be educated in order to make better health decisions. The knowledge I had gained from my upbringing did not align with the narratives to which I was exposed in school. I realized I needed to understand the foundational assumptions - theories and models – of what I was being taught. I needed to understand both their logic and their purpose, but also to find another way of telling the story of what was present in my context and is now missing in my educational stories. I needed to create and own my own narrative of my culture and place in the world.

At the time, I lacked the language to tell that story. I would later learn to appreciate the power, relevance, and nature of language as a tool of continuous improvement. I would learn that this very tool

– language – with which we must express our thoughts and soul, is the one whose mastery we still find elusive. This would lend a deeper appreciation to Toni Morrison's words captured in the expression that language may be the most important measure of our storytelling lives. To me, framing a new language of health and culture requires first that I build a new vehicle, the PEN-3 Model, and then create the path on which it could be driven, which became Health and Culture. Looking back, I see that my challenge was not only to build and refine the vehicle but also to design, construct, maintain, and keep upgrading the road. This meant going beyond the fields of public health and medicine into spaces that embraced multiple ways of telling, retelling, curating, and listening to stories, such as communications, philosophy, anthropology, psychology, history, and indeed literature. It was also a time when cultural studies were flourishing as a field, challenging orthodox ways of producing knowledge and encouraging us to question what we assumed we already knew. When it comes to language, culture shapes and nurtures how we use and understand it. Indeed, it is language that helps to make visible the place of oral tradition. In oral traditions, as the one in which I was nurtured and educated, one of the earliest skills we learn is listening, listening to allow what we hear to guide our knowing, interpretation, and engagement. It is in listening that we learn how to narrate our own stories.

Storytelling: The storyteller's most important skill is listening, and that skill is often missing in professional training spaces, especially in how we translate what we have heard into action. Growing up in Nigeria, I saw my parents as disciplined listeners, as they embodied the humility that patience and silence demand of a listener. Silence is powerful, particularly in a world filled with noise and distractions. Listening means sitting in and with stories, even when their meanings are not immediately clear, trusting that they may return later with deeper appreciation, insights, and significance. Listening is an active voice, and it is never about being muted. It is about cultivating the skill of being attentive to others' voices while also processing what expressionless bodies may convey in their silence. There are different ways that I have learned to share what I learn from listening. One example is a story I shared in the 1995 edition. I shared the story of a man who found a beautiful bird, brought it home, and kept it in a cage. He was very happy with his new pet, but noticed that the bird did not share his happiness. When he asked the bird what he could do for it, the bird replied, "Open the cage." The man refused but offered to send a message to the bird's family, to let them know the bird was safe. When the man reached the bird's family and announced the situation of the bird, one of the bird's brothers collapsed, apparently dead. Shocked, the man returned home and relayed the news. Upon hearing it, the caged bird also fell over, seemingly dead. Filled with sorrow, the man opened the cage, and the bird suddenly revived and flew away, singing, "Thank you for bringing me the wisdom of my people."

This story, which I continue to cherish, is about cultural affirmation and rediscovering what we may have forgotten, especially in challenging times. It is about surfacing the lessons of the past, lessons we may have ignored or dismissed as irrelevant. Today, such lessons are part of collective efforts in times of political assault, which might include engaging in civil rights and human rights movements, or the resilience of cultures that, despite colonization and racism, not only survived but thrived. These lessons can help us understand who we are beyond what we do. The 16 scholars and practitioners whose reflections follow each chapter in this edition share similar stories, how they have drawn lessons from the past to meet the experience of the present and prepare for the future. When current political disruptions create cultural displacement, it takes our collective strength today and the wisdom of past lessons to reposition and re-anchor ourselves. This, to me, is the foundation of a cultural journey of hope.

Hope: My hope is that this new edition reinforces the commitment of those already on this journey, as represented by the interviewees' reflections, while inviting and engaging new scholars and practitioners to deepen their understanding of why we must be committed to the process as we "question the question." Many disciplines have begun to push beyond their conventional boundaries, expanding or redefining themselves. Today we have socio-epidemiologists, social demographers, and even a friend who considers himself a "social engineer," because he seeks to understand not just structures, but how people interact with them.

Looking ahead, we must acknowledge past, present, and perhaps future politically and socially disruptive times, in which the very place of culture and identity is questioned with attempts at erasure. Preparing the next generation of cultural workers and global scholars requires co-creating radical healing spaces for hope where multiple identities can find support in questioning the questions while surfacing the strength in their collectives to firmly anchor and make visible their identity and culture. We must nurture solidarity and create spaces to talk not only about the culture of some, but about the cultures of all. This principle forms the foundation for the chapter reflections in this edition.

Chapter 1

Culture, Health Promotion, and Development

THEN:

> To a large extent, culture and health coincide. Each culture gives shape to a unique *Gestalt* of health and to a unique conformation of attitudes towards pain, disease, impairment, and death, each of which designates a class of that human performance that has traditionally been called the art of suffering.
>
> *Ivan Illich,* Medical Nemesis, 1976

> The point about our development is not the supervisory transfer to us of their expertise, but our development of our own. And the way to develop Nigerian expertise is by giving ourselves the opportunity to try, fail, learn, and succeed.
>
> *Chinweizu,* Decolonizing the African Mind,1987

Culture is a system of interrelated values active enough to influence and condition perception, judgment, communication, and behavior in each society (Mazrui, 1986, p.239). Culture is as much a structure as it is economic and political, and it is rooted in institutions such as families and schools as well as in communications industries (West, 1993). When addressing the issues of identity and difference within the contexts of power, agency, and history, we must foreground the political dimensions of culture in the process of transformation (Giroux, 1994b). Culture must be understood within the context of its transformative possibilities rather than according to the unilineal measure of the West that has come to be known as *development.*

The concept of development or its ideological appropriation for Southern nations, *underdevelopment,* has been used by scholars from both Northern and Southern nations as a marker for what is considered to be an acceptable economic threshold that Southern nations must exceed in order to experience "progress." Since 1949, when Harry S Truman introduced the phrase "underdeveloped countries' into popular discourse, the hidden agenda for development has been nothing less than the Westernization of the world (for a detailed discussion of this point, see Sachs, 1992). This process has entered a new discourse at the end of the twentieth century with the valorization of *globalization*. Globalization, as a concept produced within the context of global changes, has tended to focus only on economic production, capital restructuring, and their attendant political implications, with little regard for negative cultural changes in global societies. Globalization, within health and human development constructs - like its predecessor, development - promises an acultural world, where an individual can be at home anywhere. Development concepts inherited missionary ideology: crusading to redeem converts and to "help" them get to the threshold of "progress" as defined by the West (Gronemeyer, 1992).

Unfortunately, for people in Southern nations, who make up two-thirds of the world's population, development efforts resonate with perceptions of themselves as underdeveloped, with all the pejorative connotations that it carries (Esteva, 1992). For many African countries, *development* and *progress* have come to mean growth in gross national product, even though such an equation has long been rejected by those who initiated and promoted it, including the World Bank. African development is not merely a matter of growth in GNP statistics; it is a matter of shaping certain cultural institutions, of creating and elevating critical consciousness in the African population, so that this consciousness can properly guide the production, distribution, and consumption of the items usually reflected in GNP figures (Chinweizu, Jemie, & Madubuike, 1983). The myriad positive and progressive values and mores that enabled African countries to withstand the structural violence (psychological, physical, spiritual, and cultural) of colonial as well as postcolonial oppression are being forsaken for what is believed to be the path to progress. Progress is now believed to be a natural outgrowth of development, which in turn is believed to be concomitant with modernization. *Modernization and development are touted as the twin engines of progress, even though the economic policies advanced by modernization have been incapable of addressing the transformation of the productive forces and productive relations that lead to progress.* Modernization has been nothing more than an attempt at Westernization and ideological containment of Southern nations in the name of development. Freire (1973) has observed that although development may mean modernization, not all modernization leads to development. For example, nuclear waste dumping and infant formula production continue to lead to increased morbidity and mortality, resulting in societal regression in conditions of living. This reality has become increasingly evident in assessments of the impacts and outcomes of numerous health and education programs planned for and implemented in Southern nations.

At the center of health, communication, and education initiatives is the ability to look to our past, not only for historical continuity but for understanding about the trials, failures, and possibilities that shape our individual and collective experiences. "We affirm the ties of the past, the bonds of the present, when we relearn our history, nurture the shared sensibility that has been retained in the present, linking these gestures to resistance struggle, to liberation movements that seek to eradicate domination and transform society" (hooks, 1992, p.194). As Stuart Hall (1991) notes, the relation that people of the world have to their own past is a part of the discovery and affirmation of their own ethnicity: "The past is not only a position from which to speak, but it is also an absolutely necessary resource in what one has to say" (p.18). These past and present experiences constitute a group's cultural identity.

Cultural identity is based primarily on shared historical, linguistic, and psychological lineage (Diop, 1991). These sets of collective factors in a culture influence the group's design for living, the shared set of socially transmitted perceptions about the nature of the physical, social, and spiritual world, particularly as it relates to achieving life's goals (Basch, 1990). As Henry Giroux (1992) observes, culture "is not an object of unquestioning reverence but a mobile field of ideological and material relations that are unfinished, multilayered, and always open to interrogation" (p. 99). "Culture embodies those moral, ethical, and aesthetic values, the set of spiritual eyeglasses, through which people come to view themselves and their place in the universe. Language as a culture is the collective memory bank of a people's experience in history" (Thiong'O, 1993, p.14). Those who develop health and education programs must examine carefully the differences as well as the similarities in cultural perceptions, to understand health beliefs and practices more fully and to address them appropriately within their contexts. Such understanding should not be based on market economy and buying power, the traditional indices of development. Culture evolves and is sustained within the process of a people wrestling with the natural and social environment, and thus embodies the moral, aesthetic, and ethical values that are manifested in the people's consciousness (Thiong'O, 1993).

Important aspects of cultural expression in African countries are found in aesthetic values and meanings, as evident in arts, music, and clothing. Such values and meanings are laden with desires, emotions, and expectations that may not be discernible through Westernized code. For example, "the notion of religion is hardly ever used [by Westerners] to designate African beliefs and religious practices" (Mudimbe, 1988, p.76). In an attempt to show "the ways things really are" in the non-West, we have become engaged in discourses that produce a non-West that is deprived of fantasy, desires, and contradictory emotions (Chow, 1991). It is the omission of these aesthetic values from the analytic framework used to examine African cultures that renders external approaches to African experience Eurocentric. Marxist literary criticism is limited by its insistence on the tendency to base aesthetic assessment solely on how the market economy shapes the political struggle of the proletariat. This market-driven analysis tends to make Marxist literary criticism thin on what are commonly considered aesthetic concerns in African traditions, thus ignoring, or denouncing as "formalism," questions of beauty, style, technique, sensibility, and appropriateness, which are at the core of African aesthetics (Chinweizu, 1987).

In public health, health promotion and behavior change programs, "cultural sensitivity" refers to the need to develop programs in ways that are consistent with a people's and community's cultural framework, rather than based on the Western paradigm within which most health, education, and development programs are planned, implemented, and evaluated. Health denotes a process of adaptation. It is the result not of instinct, but of an autonomous yet culturally shaped reaction to socially created reality (Illich, 1976). For example, illness is a socially recognized state, carrying with it certain specific drawbacks, obligations, and privileges, depending on the circumstances (Basch, 1990). Each culture creates its own responses to health and disease. For the same symptoms - of kleptomania, for example - in different cultures, an individual might be executed, sentenced to death, exiled, hospitalized, or given arms or tax money (Illich, 1976).

The Discourse of Difference in Health and Education

Eurocentric approaches to global educational processes should be deconstructed and reconstructed to reflect varied cultural expressions. Attempts to affirm cultural differences in schools and communities often manifest themselves in calls for program and curriculum integration, although program/curriculum reformation/transformation is a more progressive approach to centralizing diversity in the learning process. In some cases, special programs are developed to redress the grievances of the marginalized. Racism is often atoned for through measures aimed at eliminating racist institutional barriers in the marketplace and through the provision of compensatory programs to enhance the cultural capital and skills of the oppressed, as has been evident in various remedial programs designed for African Americans in schools and the workplace (Giroux, 1992).

In a culture-centered approach to health, education, and communication, the experiences of the Others must be centralized in the mainstream school curriculum for the benefit of students from both the center and the margin. "To open up to the culture's soul is to allow one to become wet, to become soaked in the cultural and historical waters of those individuals who are involved in the experience" (Freire, 1993, p.106). Such involvement and total commitment are transformative for both the interventionists and the target population. The resulting reformation of the curriculum/programmatic paradigm includes affirmation and encouragement of different languages of expression, health beliefs, and cultural values. For example, binary opposition is unnecessarily constructed between modern information channels that are based on the Western construct and traditional information channels (oral communication). Both systems of communication are effectively functional within their contexts; in some cases, the two are quite complementary. Unfortunately, many health communication programs in the past have negated a form of cultural production by ignoring oral communication. This has been true particularly in the planning, implementation, and evaluation of programs in many African cultures. Ngugi Wa Thiong'O (1993) notes that the biggest weapon wielded and unleashed daily by imperialism against the oppressed and the exploited of the earth is the cultural bomb:

> The effect of a cultural bomb is to annihilate a people's belief in their names, in their languages, in their environment, in their heritage of struggle, in their unity, in their capacities, and ultimately in themselves. It makes them see their past as one wasteland of non-achievement, and it makes them want to distance themselves from the wasteland. (p. 3)

Ultimately, a broader discourse on the politics of representation in health promotion calls for the decolonization of the minds of the members of the marginalized group. Africans, Asians, Latin Americans, as well as African Americans and members of other U.S. minority groups, must insist on appropriate representation in the production of knowledge and cultural identity, particularly concerning learning opportunities in health and development. Although some interventionists understand and respect the value of oral tradition, the programmatic response to this form of cultural expression tends to focus only on the storyteller. This is consistent with classical pedagogy, which positions the teacher/educator as the ultimate repository of knowledge and relegates students to the status of objects that cannot produce knowledge but can only acquire it. Ultimately, the teacher/ educator is disempowered by the failure to engage the learner in the co-creation of knowledge such that the terrain of learning is multiaccented and mutually enriching. In an attempt to construct what they believe to be a terrain of learning for the voiceless, interventionists assume the role of the storyteller by constructing stories under the guise of cultural sensitivity. Such an approach fails to understand the dynamic of the story listener, which is equally important as, if not more important than, that of the storyteller.

Cultural dynamics such as communication codes, meanings, and context between the storyteller and listener promote knowledge production and acquisition. Thus, oral tradition generally is not only the heritage of the spoken or sung word; it is also the heritage of the ear (Faseke, 1990). Stated differently, people in oral traditional cultures (as in many African countries) are accustomed to learning by listening. Learning by seeing is important to the extent that what is seen is congruent with what is heard. Critical aspects of learning by listening include *who* was speaking, the way the words were expressed, and in what context. This issue raises questions about the ethical and cultural incongruence of assuming the role of storyteller without training or education for that role, and without a thorough understanding of the cultural implications of storytelling for learning. I do not mean to generalize here about all African cultures as cultures of the ear; rather, I want to emphasize the importance of taking this form of cultural expression into account in health intervention projects as a valued form and sometimes the primary form of cultural production. Storytelling requires that one immerse oneself in the storytelling tradition, undergo an appropriate apprenticeship, master the verbal arts, and be able to write one's own re-creations of traditional stories (Chinweizu et al., 1983). The storyteller, through whom truth is summoned to unwind itself to the audience, is a creator, a delighter, and a teacher (Minh-ha, 1991).

Given the realities of cultural production, we can conclude that the use of posters, flyers, and other pictorial learning tools in health promotion and health communication programs may have limited, if any, impact in many cultures. Even when such materials are culturally appropriate, there are still questions to be addressed with respect to when and how they should be used. Alternative methods of cross-cultural communication should be explored to ensure that the process does not disempower the target group. *When listening is the culturally appropriate method of learning, health, communication, and education professionals involved in developing, implementing, and evaluating programs in cultures other than their own should be required to develop the requisite skills for effective and meaningful program implementation for listening.* Furthermore, institutions of higher learning that have claimed intellectual hegemony over teaching and learning should reform their health curricula to reflect the cultural realities of the global population. Chapter 2 addresses the role of culture in communication, particularly as it relates to health information and beliefs.

NOW:

My conversation with Bunmi Makinwa and Davison Munodawafa

Cultural and Professional Identity - Positionality

Airhihenbuwa: I identify as a father, husband, uncle, elder, brother, teacher, friend, and student. Culturally and ethnically, I'm an Edo man rooted in Edo (Nigerian) culture. Racially, I'm a Black man in America, anchored in contemporary African American experiences. Professionally, I'm located at the intersection of health, communication, language, and identity. These are the lenses through which I understand culture at a broader level, and they define my professional space. I don't fit neatly into a single academic discipline, rather, my contributions are informed by multiple cultural and intellectual actors from spaces that reflect both who I am and the communities I serve.

Makinwa: I primarily see myself as an African, more specifically, a Nigerian, deeply rooted in the African way of life. Both my education and professional journey have taken me across many African countries, enriching my identity and understanding. At the same time, I've been fortunate to be closely connected with the Western world, especially through my academic and professional experiences. I often say I stand with one foot in Africa and one foot in the West, which allows me to see both the linkages and contrasts across these cultural spheres. Professionally, I'm a retired behavioral communication practitioner. I didn't follow a purely academic path, instead, I was deeply involved in applying communication strategies to understand social, community, and individual behaviors, especially as they relate to health. What's been most meaningful to me is collaborating with others, like both of you, in striving to bring an African lens to health behavior analysis. Now in retirement, I dedicate more time to writing and offering advisory support.

Munodawafa: Culturally, I see myself first and foremost as an African, with my identity anchored especially in Southern Africa. I recognize the nuanced differences across the continent, between North, East, West, and Southern Africa, but my experience and sense of self have been most influenced by the Southern region. In my retirement, I've been reflecting on a role I probably played unknowingly for years, as a bridge or conveyor belt within the African context.

The Place of Culture in Your Professional Journeys

Airhihenbuwa: What was your journey like even before retirement and now in retirement, especially considering what the chapter addresses, the dominance of Western perspectives in defining development?

Makinwa: The issue you raised in the chapter, how development has been defined primarily through a Western paradigm, applies not only to development but across many domains. In fact, history itself is filled with interpretations shaped by the worldview of the writer. The writer becomes a conveyor, carrying what is on the belt. But if the belt is empty, the conveyor delivers nothing. For there to be a story, there must be something on that belt. So, writers, interpreters, and analysts define narratives based on their contexts, be it in history, politics, economics, development, or health. Objectivity, then, is always filtered through one's own lens. I think, therefore I am. But even that thinking, *Cogito, ergo sum*, takes place within the limits of what one knows, what one has experienced, and the concepts one has access to. As we acquired knowledge, many of us began to see that the frameworks we were taught, especially those from Western paradigms, did not always align with the lived realities of our own communities. The education we received, from elementary through to college, was thoroughly Western. But as we advanced, we began to critically examine that education, questioning its assumptions, its definitions, and how it framed us.

Fortunately, alternative viewpoints began to emerge. We encountered literature that reflected our own cultures or other non-Western perspectives, offering paradigms that made more sense in our contexts. *We began to balance both worldviews, Western and African, recognizing that development exists in our cultures too, though it may not be expressed through material symbols like scientific instruments or modern infrastructure.* Instead, development could mean social cohesion, adaptability, or the ingenuity to thrive under difficult conditions.

This critical awakening also reshaped our understanding of health. That's when I began to read your work, Airhihenbuwa, as you compellingly argued for the centrality of culture in understanding and promoting health. Your work helped us see that our cultural frameworks were not obstacles but powerful tools, tools for self-understanding, for integration, and for overcoming health challenges. When we worked with UNAIDS on HIV/AIDS, we realized how crucial it was to consider the whole person and their community, not just their symptoms. In the early years, there was no treatment or cure for HIV. This forced us to explore other ways of responding to the crisis, ways rooted in culture, dignity, and community. And that shift was only possible because we stepped outside the Western paradigm and embraced our own.

Munodawafa: I spent much of my early and professional life outside Zimbabwe, leaving in 1983 and returning in 2017. I lived and worked in the U.S., India, Congo-Brazzaville, and other places. Each location shaped how I saw myself and how others expected me to be. *Language has always been central to my expression of identity.* In Zimbabwe, for example, I speak both Shona and Ndebele as a way to reaffirm my Africanness. Professionally, I'm an educator by training and passion. I began as a nurse and later pursued advanced degrees in public health, with a focus on health promotion and community engagement. Communication is at the heart of my work, understanding how people receive, process, and use health information is a key concern for me. Though I'm officially retired, I've returned to the classroom, now teaching in a medical school. It's a new and exciting space for me, having previously focused on public health education. I teach students from their first year all the way through to their final year, and I love it.

Past Lessons on Health and Development Solutions in Africa

Airhihenbuwa: Makinwa, you mentioned the UNAIDS HIV and AIDS Communication Framework, which you initiated. I noted during the 30th anniversary webinar of this book that you were among the first to invite me to Nairobi to discuss the book. You gathered a diverse group of African professionals engaged in development communication across various UN and non-UN agencies. Could you speak to that experience, especially as someone trained as a journalist who later assumed a senior leadership role in the UN? You previously described the writer as someone who interprets the story.

Makinwa: I joined WHO earlier on at a leadership level as head of information for Africa at the regional office in Brazzaville. However, the hierarchy there meant that every decision, even for a budget that was technically yours, had to pass through multiple approvals, culminating with the regional director. Often, your funds would be reallocated despite being designated for your initiatives. This inefficiency and bureaucracy pushed me to leave WHO after just two years, convinced I would never work within the UN system. But over time, I realized a vital lesson: when you are in a leadership role that includes budgetary control, much can be achieved, even within a bureaucratic system. So, I returned to UNAIDS with my eyes wide open, this time as the head of global communication. With control over my budget, I could bring in global perspectives, from Asia, Latin America, Europe, and Africa, to shape a new mindset on HIV prevention. At the time, there was no treatment or control for HIV. Prevention was the only path forward. But HIV was laden with stigma, viewed by some as a sexual or even divine punishment. To effectively address it, we had to understand people's worldviews.

We asked: How have people historically survived enormous challenges? What spiritual, cultural, and social logic shapes their response? We drew insights from scholars like you and colleagues from around the world, understanding that people approach health with cultural lenses, whether African, Asian, or Latin American.

These lenses reflect their economic, spiritual, and social lives, which in turn shape health decisions. That insight led to what you, Airhihenbuwa, describe in his book as a cultural interpretation of health, how people use their cultural frameworks to confront or cope with serious challenges.

Of course, this wasn't without resistance. We were introducing new approaches in a space long dominated by established organizations like the WHO and UNICEF. We weren't asking them to abandon their methods but to consider additional, culturally grounded perspectives. Fortunately, UNAIDS, as a secretariat to various UN bodies, gave us the platform to involve these organizations diplomatically and respectfully. We included accomplished professionals, yourselves among them, who resonated with our approach. Over time, WHO, UNICEF, and many others became active contributors to the UNAIDS HIV Communication Framework. Ultimately, holding a leadership position with budgetary authority made all the difference. It gave me the means, the voice, and the platform to speak boldly and catalyze meaningful change.

Training the Next Generation

Airhihenbuwa: As you, Munodawafa, reflect on the next phase of this journey, imagine the younger generation, whether students, practitioners, or members of community-based organizations, looking to you for guidance. What should they focus on? How should they think about identity in the context of these challenges?

Munodawafa: Before joining WHO, I spent five years in Malawi helping to establish a quasi-UN agency called the Guidance, Counseling, and Youth Development Centre for Africa. Supported by UNESCO, this Center was created under the auspices of African Ministers of Education. It emerged in response to the devastating impact of the HIV and AIDS pandemic on children and youth across the continent and began operations in 2000. We organized summer trainings for teachers from various African countries, focusing on guidance, counseling, and life skills development, drawing from both UNICEF and UNESCO frameworks. As the Center's first Executive Director, my mandate was to broaden its focus beyond

HIV/AIDS. We introduced initiatives addressing racism in South African schools, promoted harmony, launched entrepreneurship programs, and addressed mental health concerns.

Looking ahead, we must confront the growing severity of drug abuse and the spread of more potent alcohol among youth in countries like Zimbabwe, Zambia, and Malawi. Issues surrounding adolescent's sexual health are also escalating. These trends call for differentiated, multi-level interventions within school systems. The COVID-19 pandemic was a wake-up call. With schools closed for up to two years in some regions, institutions realized the necessity of building stronger ties with their surrounding communities and preparing for future health emergencies. Technology has also taken center stage. Tools like mobile phones, once prohibited, became essential for delivering instruction during school closures, revealing their critical role in future education strategies. There is an urgent need for a paradigm shift toward preventative care and primary healthcare, especially given the continent's technological and infrastructural limitations. I would advocate for focusing on cultural practices in nutrition to enhance health outcomes and ease the burden on hospitals, encouraging health professionals to prioritize prevention over reactive medical intervention.

Final Thoughts

There is an urgent need to advance cultural approaches to development and healthcare in resource-limited settings. This was the central message of the chapter when it was first written 30 years ago, and it remains relevant today. We must challenge the prevailing mindset in international development to better maximize limited resources. Prevention continues to be the cornerstone of improving health in African and other Southern nations. The conversation concludes with reflections on how to leverage geopolitical turbulence as a moment to reassess development strategies, especially considering the recent restructuring of the WHO into three main clusters: health systems, health promotion and prevention, and health emergencies.

Chapter 2

Communicating Health Within Culture

THEN:

> I do not believe that the mass media change people's attitudes and beliefs, but I believe that learning experiences do. The mass media are influential in so far as they are, or can be, part of good learning experiences.
>
> *Andreas Fuglesang,* Applied Communication in Developing Countries,1973

Cultural codes, symbols, and values embody the essence of meaning that people bring to the production and acquisition of knowledge. These forms of cultural expression are accented in the meanings that participants bring to the communication of health messages. The dialogic process necessarily accents verbal and non-verbal exchange such that participants' behaviors are culturally meaningful.

Health, Communication, and Education professionals and others who design health promotion and disease prevention programs must examine health behaviors in particular cultures in terms of whether they are rooted in the cultural values and beliefs of the people. For example, it has been demonstrated that in several African countries, person-to-person communication (through home visits) has been more effective in changing negative health behaviors than having messages distributed through the mass media. This finding is undoubtedly related to the oral tradition that is the customary bedrock for the co-creation and acquisition of knowledge, as well as the construction of reality, in African cultures. Educating students and audiences serves as an introduction to how a culture is organized, a demonstration of who should speak for whom, and what within the culture is considered invalid and unworthy of public recognition (Giroux, 1992).

Health Promotion and Cultural Communication

If the bullet is the means of physical subjugation, language is the means of spiritual subjugation (Thiong'O, 1986). Fuglesang (1973) concludes that the most effective method of learning is through demonstration, because the learner uses all the senses - hearing, smell, vision, taste, and touch. Unfortunately, most of the health communication programs that have been implemented in Southern nations have emphasized only visual learning. Fuglesang also notes that visual literacy is an acquired skill.

Central to the issue of cultural variance in the production and acquisition of knowledge (as discussed in Chapter 1) is how the notion of visual literacy as a "superior form of learning" devalues orature and orality, as theorized and practiced in many African countries, as forms of cultural production. Seeing and/or visualizing, as expressed in such idioms as "You see what I mean" and "Get the picture?" are more symbolic of mental imagery than of visual learning, although visualizing can serve as a reinforcer. The notion of knowledge co-creation and acquisition through what one sees suggests a physical vision as opposed to a mental vision. Mental vision has transformative possibilities that should be promoted in oral cultures such as those found in many African societies.

In societies in which cultural production is realized primarily through orality, the ability to engage in the production of individual and collective mental imagery in learning is superior to visual/physical abilities. This process of cultural communication is eschewed in many health programs being implemented today in most African countries. Instead of focusing on encouraging the production of mental vision that engages individuals by affirming their own space and voice, institutions of higher learning (which, for the most part, provide training instead of education), as well as development agencies, have naturalized and reified the production of standardized learning based on physical vision. The result is a push for physical learning, such as the use of audiovisuals like PowerPoints (as opposed to transparencies and slide projectors in previous generations), as the ultimate form of sharing and communicating knowledge based culturally on philosophy and practice. In fact, some institutions in both Northern and Southern nations have gone so far as to require that those who share knowledge, whether students making classroom presentations or professionals presenting conference papers, use physical/visual materials as the primary tool of communication, with the speaker's voice serving only a secondary function.

This form of learning has been promoted even though very few educators and communicators can effectively and efficiently use and update their skills in these audiovisuals and related tools to engage their audiences in the production and acquisition of knowledge. For the majority, such presentations have become a form of standardized mediocrity; the speaker no longer has to aspire toward acquiring a voice that can transport the audience and/or student to undertake an independent cultural journey that leads to the production of meaning. Rather, professionals have settled for a uniform, often Western- and male-centered meaning - the ultimate form of what Freire (1973) refers to as "castration of curiosity" in learners. The paradox in this case becomes evident in how we reward speakers and affirm leadership in education. In certain circumstances, it is the individual who can "stand and deliver," in the absence of visual support, who is worthy of recognition. Evidence of this tradition abounds among people of African descent.

> The scholar, rhetorician, or historian who undertakes an analysis of the Black past without recognizing the significance of vocal expression as a transforming agent is treading on intellectual quicksand... What is clear is that leaders who articulated and articulate the grievances felt by the masses have always understood the power of the word in the Black community... Their emergence has always been predicated upon the power of the spoken word. (Asante, 1987, p. 86)

The power of the spoken word has always been recognized by Africans as the hallmark of the varied interpretations and value of storytelling. Such interpretations are sometimes encoded in songs of a story, such that the wisdom of the story is recalled in the song. *The Edos of Nigeria* always begin a story by singing a song that captures the spirit and the message of the story. Songs and dances are central to nearly all Edo rituals celebrating birth, rain, marriage, the *Igue festival,* as well as funerals and more conventional ceremonies. Songs and dances are not just decorative additions to an occasion; they are an integral part of the conversation, the drinking session, the ritual, the ceremony (Thiong'O, 1986).

Although songs and dances are central to the Edo form of cultural production, individuals need certain skills to navigate the terrain of meanings and codes enshrined in the cultural landscape. Such skills are often acquired through experiential education and training. Indifferent and sometimes oblivious to the significance of songs and dances, as well as storytelling, in many African countries, Westernized/Eurocentric intellectuals have often engaged themselves in these media of expression even though they have no training, skills, or understanding of these forms of cultural production. Such culture-effacing acts are an extension of the belief that orature/oracy as a form of cultural production is simplistic, premodern, and easily engaged in by anyone with basic training in the more "complex" (written tradition) form of cultural production. Untrained and inexperienced in oral communication and acting from their incorrect perceptions of the simplicity of the oral genre, these individuals produce simple stories and songs that defy cultural codes, interpretations, and meanings. Chinweizu, Jemie, and Madubuike (1983), in their classic book *Toward the Decolonization of African Literature*, challenge the prejudices that are often espoused by Eurocentrists when evaluating African literature and oral tradition:

> In evaluating African literature and matters related to it, they [Eurocentrists] start out by taking outstanding written material from Europe as their standards; they gather whatever African material they find convenient, usually of middling quality or worse, and compare them adversely with the best from Europe,

> and thereby unctuously confirm themselves in their initial prejudice that Europe is "good" and Africa is "bad." When it comes to the African oral tradition, their anti-African prejudice is reinforced by their anti-oral prejudice. They therefore gather the most grossly inadequate versions of African oral material they can find, and proceed, once again, to unctuously confirm themselves in their double-barreled prejudice against things both African and oral. (p.87)

The use of language in any culture is designed to mirror the worldview of the culture. It is often suggested that African languages have limitations in their usage, but this is a myopic conclusion that uses Western standards to evaluate the lexical functions of all languages and their cultural relevancies. According to Chinweizu et al. (1983), the "issue of parity and reciprocity has implications for the matter of making comparisons between the oral and written modes. Cognizance ought to be taken of the diversity of genres within the oral and the written forms, so that only comparable forms are compared" (p. 35). The possibilities of the oral genre include the mystification of reality and the reality of myths, the spontaneity of communication and communicating spontaneously, and the extension of the interpretive potentials of cultural codes and meanings, even when invoked for the first time.

A common theme in the stories of African cultures is the interaction between animate and inanimate objects. This has been demonstrated in the fictional works of Wole Soyinka and Ben Okri, among others, in which people assume animal functions and roles and vice versa. Trees and other inanimate objects can communicate verbally. Earthly phenomena, such as animal forms and their peculiarities, are explained in fables.

Knowledge is culturally produced through forms of direct and indirect exchange between parents and children, teachers and students, and speakers and audiences. For example, the colonial mentality of expecting non-Western cultures to embrace Western paradigms without critically analyzing them creates a lose/lose situation. To suggest that non-Western cultures should play a catch-up game with the West is to suggest that their cultural values and production could never equate with "progress." Meanwhile, the West continues to devise new markers for "progress," from *savage* to *underdevelopment/development*, and now *globalization*.

This relationship of the West to the rest of us can be illustrated by the relationship between the egg and the coconut - it does not matter whether the egg falls on the coconut or the coconut falls on the egg, it is the egg that will break. The coconut and egg represent different identities that, allowing for some possibilities of hybridization, in principle affirm each other's space. Considered side by side, they represent different forms of cultural production and meaning on the global landscape. They echo the philosophy that searches for multiple truths because when one thing stands, another thing stands beside it. Neither the egg nor the coconut is static in its cultural representation. In other words, whereas a culture may symbolize the egg in one instance, in another it may be the coconut. For example, although many African cultural codes and meanings (the coconut) were impervious to assault during colonialism and postcolonialism (i.e., the introduction of traditional medicine), these same societies have yielded (the egg) to the adoption and often valorization of non-African languages for political, educational, personal, and business/market exchanges. By the same token, although the Western cultures have maintained their religious traditions (the coconut), these same cultures have yielded (the egg) some formal codes and are now being influenced by music (such as Raps and Afrobeats) and clothing constructed by African Americans and Africans.

The victor in the cultural clash of such forms of knowledge acquisition becomes a part of a culture and establishes the initial basis upon which subsequent opinions are formulated, attitudes and values developed, new inquisitions made, and new knowledge produced. The use of adages and proverbs is usually the hallmark of changes in educational training and cultural codes in traditional settings. It is very important for the rest of us to understand the full ramifications of undue reliance on Western paradigms for the meaning of progress. There are long-term, irreversible consequences for continuing to operate under Western hegemonic influences, because, as my mother always reminded us as children, "no one said a child should not have big teeth as long as s/he has lips big enough to cover them." For example, in 1973, Robert McNamara, president of the World Bank, declared that GNP as a singular measure of development has exacerbated inequalities in income distribution, because more and more people become poorer as GNP grows (Illich, 1992). In other words, development as conceived in the West has led to regression in the standard of living in Southern nations.

Two decades after the realization of the failure of the development concept, and four years after the U.N. Development Programme's (1993) *Human Development Report* called for the inclusion and emphasis of noneconomic indicators (e.g., food security and status of women) in measuring progress, the implementation of the development concept as informed by the dominant paradigm continues to flourish in Southern nations. Although World Bank and U.N. Development Programme reports have questioned the validity of equating development/GNP with progress, they have still failed to centralize cultural production and meaning at the core of the measurement of progress.

If the importance of a cultural domain affects the lexical complexity of that domain, then the absence of words to delineate family kinship along biological lines in many African cultures is of lexical significance. According to W. Kamau (personal communication, 1993), among the Kikuyus of Kenya, the first male child (I do not say "first son" because the terms *son* and *daughter* resonate with parent-child closure that does not allow for the inclusion of other members of the extended family in the rearing of the child) bears the name of his paternal grandfather and the first female child bears the name of the paternal grandmother. The second male child bears the name of the maternal grandfather, and the second female child bears the name of the maternal grandmother. The relationships that exist between children and grandparents in this context are rooted in a strong belief that the future (our children) is an extension of the past (our parents). A grandparent becomes closely bonded with his or her rebirth (the grandchild) and assumes unflinching and unwavering personal responsibility toward the child. The child is often referred to in the name and designation of his or her grandparent, whose life the child is on earth to relive. The child soon begins to internalize the role, persona, and values of the grandparent in a psychologically preordained role-modeling relationship. In most cases, according to Kamau, the child begins to manifest certain physical and behavioral traits of the grandparent - a powerful form of family and cultural reproduction.

Among the Kikuyus, these cultural codes and meanings are critical for couples' decisions regarding the number of children they desire (a goal for family planning programs) and the number of children they have in the process of seeking to balance the gender representations of the children as a fulfillment of their cultural expressions. Such cultural fulfillment may result in undue pressure on a couple, especially the wife, to have at least two boys and two girls. However, the bonding, psychogenealogical extension, and family and cultural reproductions are values and nurturing that symbiotically benefit the children and parents in their collective growth and transformation. These collective experiences, which are not always quantifiable - nor should they be - are the hallmark of the sustenance of the extended family in Africa.

The fact that many relatives are referred to as brothers and sisters (even though these include those who would be considered nephews, nieces, and cousins in Western cultures) is often believed to be an example of the limitations of languages in African cultures. The possibility that this way of languaging kinships is deliberately constructed to capture the closeness and bonding that typifies the sibling relationship is rarely entertained. To learn that there is a difference between one's brothers/sisters and one's cousins and other so-called distant relations is to learn about developing cognitive and affective distance in the way one relates to those relatives. Among the Edos of Nigeria, where children are familiar only with the concept of brothers and sisters, there is a type of closeness and reciprocal responsibility peculiar to the culture that is theirs to value. In fact, the concept of brothers and sisters in the African context is one of the most important factors in the maintenance and sustenance of the extended family in Africa.

Moreover, the term *extended family* suggests that the Westernized nuclear family is the norm. When the extended family is used as the norm, situating it at the center instead of the margin, the Western family becomes the alternative type of family, the "constricted family." When I was growing up in Nigeria, I always knew that my nephew was my brother. Upon coming to the United States for "training," I began to refer to my brother by the Western designation (my nephew). As time progressed, I began to experience some level of inexplicable mental distance that was never the case in Nigeria. It was as though I suddenly discovered that my brother was adopted by my parents, but unfortunately, my parents were not with me to buffer the shock and confusion that followed this discovery. It was up to me alone to overcome the irrelevance of the Western genealogical demarcation, as it were, and hold on to the wisdom of my parents and my culture. I had to make a conscious effort to revert to referring to my brother as my brother.

I would argue that our forebears intentionally left out words and delineators that could potentially distance relatives. Such cultural wealth and vision affirm and speak to the cultural strength, sophistication, and pragmatism of Africans in the co-production of knowledge, with its carefully constructed cultural codes and meanings. Of course, for Eurocentrists, to affirm this is to subscribe to an episteme that is not consistent with or may be superior to that of the West. One does not have to understand or logically follow cultural codes or expressions to affirm and respect their legitimating values. After all, everyday language usage that defies logic has always influenced the interpretive meanings and visual imagery given to life experience. For example, we speak of *sunrise* and *sunset*, although these terms tend to suggest that the world is flat rather than that the Earth spins in its orbit around the sun. This has never stopped people from using these expressions or led them to change their value and meaning, even though perhaps more accurate terms would be *earthrise* and *earthset.*

Cultural practices relating to patterns of knowledge production and acquisition, in this case oral tradition, must be seriously considered in health communication interventions in cultures in which orature is the primary basis of communication. Health communication projects conducted in Africa to date have tended to operate on three key assumptions:

1. Health information can reach the populace through the media.

2. This health information can change negative health practices if the population has the requisite health knowledge. Therefore, the health information should focus on the acquisition of the relevant health knowledge.

3. If the people do not acquire the relevant health information, it means that their skills for acquiring this information must be developed. This often translates to the development of literacy programs for the population. In fact, literacy is being hailed as the key to improving the health conditions of Africans.

The problem with these operational assumptions is that they place all of the responsibility for program outcomes on the actions or inaction of the people in the communities. Therefore, if a program fails, it is always reasoned that the target community lacked the requisite knowledge and/or motivation to initiate the expected health actions that would lead to positive health outcomes. The health communication interventionists are absolved of any responsibility and accountability for the failure of the program participants to attain the expected health outcomes. Eurocentrists refuse to interrogate their complicity in the formation and imposition of their cultural hegemony on Others as constructed in the interplay of language and difference (Giroux, 1992). One of the manifestations of this interplay is the proliferation of adult literacy programs in Africa.

Literacy and Educational Interventions

Unfortunately, literacy has been equated with education and, ultimately, stages and levels of development. Although literacy is usually a by-product of Western formal education, education (skills coupled with experience to make informed decisions) is not always the outcome of literacy. In fact, some of the traditional literacy programs were designed to provide unsuspecting consumers with the skills to understand and purchase certain commercially advertised products. This is not surprising, given that literacy is believed to be the springboard to national development.

The misguided notion of literacy as a precursor for national development is based on Anderson's (1966) claim that a society requires a 40% adult literacy rate for economic "takeoff" (cited in Street, 1984). This paradigm has resulted in the widespread development and promotion of adult literacy programs, particularly in Southern nations. This practice continues today, even though people tend to lose literacy skills if their daily engagements do not involve reading and/or writing. In fact, several of the illiterate adults in some African countries today were once able to read and write as a result of completing primary school education. The ability to read and write is like many other skills in that you can learn it, but if you do not use it, you lose it. Thus, most of the current literacy programs are simply reinventing the wheel - or, worse yet, they are reinventing the flat tire.

UNESCO attempted to improve the sustainability of literacy skills by creating what it called a "literacy environment" (Street, 1984). This simply meant that the environment of a community would be transformed to fit the needs and desires of those promoting the literacy program, rather than the program being modified to fit with the community environment. Challenging UNESCO and others who perpetrate this neocolonial violence on Southern nations, Freire (1973) and some other cultural workers proposed adult literacy programs that engage the participants as subjects rather than objects. Using this approach, participants are engaged in the construction of sociopolitical issues that shape their collective reality, in a "process of *conscienciization*." In Freire's adult literacy model, the participants are exposed to social and political issues that affect them so that they can become involved and have input into the decisions that affect them. "No program of literacy-training can exist - as the naive claim - which is not connected with the work of human beings, their technical proficiency, their view of the world" (Freire, 1973, p.157), because "literacy involves not just the reading of the word, but also the reading of the World" (Freire, 1993, p. 59).

Even when the goal of a literacy program is sensitive to the cultural reality of the people the program is designed to benefit, the methods and techniques of implementation are often not culturally sensitive. In this respect, it is important to examine the methods employed in health communications. Specifically, we should examine the level of congruence between the traditional mode of learning (oral - mouth to ear) and the Western mode of learning (visual - eye to object). In other words, to what degree does the use of posters and flyers, which are visually dependent, conflict with the traditional method of learning in an oral tradition? Literacy is critical to the degree that it problematizes the very structure and practice of representation by focusing attention on the fact that meaning is not fixed and that to be literate is to undertake a dialogue with others who speak from different histories, locations, and experiences (Giroux, 1992). Literacy is yet another development index that has been used to pursue the notion of universal truths.

A major problem in the planning and development of health, education, and communication programs has been the preoccupation with seeking a universal solution. This fixation has resulted in the misrepresentation of the diverse cultural realities of Africans, as though they are monolithic. As Freire (1970) notes:

> One of the characteristics of oppressive cultural action, which is almost never perceived by the dedicated but naive professionals who are involved, is the emphasis on a focalized view of problems rather than on seeing them as dimensions of a totality. In "community development" projects the more a region or area is broken down into "local communities," without the study of these communities both as totalities in themselves and as part of another totality (the area, region, and so forth) - which in its turn is a part of a still larger totality (the nation, as part of the continental totality) - the more alienation is intensified. (p.138)

On the issue of universal truth espoused in the dominant paradigm, Faundez comments, "Whereas Europeans try to discover what there is in *common*, and that becomes the essential for them, for me the essential is the `differences,' and, since each time I discover differences, each time I become more aware of how little I know" (in Freire & Faundez, 1989, p. 32).

As a consultant to the World Health Organization in 1991, I was asked to develop a health education curriculum in Geneva (this request did not come from the Division of Health Education). This guideline was to be used in the development of health curricula in several African countries, without the involvement of participants from those countries. I protested and registered my objection to being a party to a process that totally disempowers the teachers, administrators, and students in these countries. Such is a Geneva hegemony (in spite of the fact that some WHO programs tend to be progressive) that marginalizes Africans by denying them the opportunity to be subjects and actors in the systematization of educational processes that will shape their future. This sophisticated form of colonization is practiced by using a credentialed member of the marginalized group to sustain Western hegemony in the name of inclusion and pluralism. *It has become a common practice for national and international institutions to recruit unsuspecting credentialed Others (including Third World nationals and members of minority groups in the First World) to pursue and promote what are believed to be universal solutions to the problems of the 'Others'.* Although an increase in the representation and involvement of disenfranchised Others is welcome, it does not absolve decision makers of their responsibility to examine their complicitous actions/inactions and myopic approaches. Neither should these practices continue to exclude the participation of Others in the production of knowledge and cultural identity.

Conclusion

Cultural sensitivity in health, education, communication, and development programs can be realized only when we centralize the cultural experiences of those who have hitherto been marginalized in the production of knowledge and cultural identity. To be specific, it is counterproductive to target individuals for most health risk reduction efforts without considering the effects of those individuals' cultures, languages, and environments. Educators must draw on expertise at a location to address the social, political, and environmental forces that influence health behavior within the context of particular cultures (Airhihenbuwa, DiClemente, Wingood, & Lowe, 1992). However, the onus of transforming these environmental forces must not rest solely on the people targeted for health promotion and disease prevention. Ultimately, the source experts are catalysts; they must be seen as symbolic of the resolve and potential of the groups they represent, not as exceptions. The true experts in the methods of the production and acquisition of knowledge in a culture are the people themselves. In Chapter 3, I present a cultural model and examples of its application to various population groups.

NOW:

My Conversation with Rafael Obregon and Khadidiatou Ndiaye

Cultural and Professional Identity - Positionality

Airhihenbuwa: I repeated my intro in Chapter One.

Ndiaye: Culturally, I identify as a proud Muslim Senegalese woman and a member of the *Ndiath*, a term that may be Westernized in spelling but holds deep traditional roots. I am a wife, an aunt, and a member of a large family. I also identify, somewhat reluctantly, with hybrid cultures. I've spent more of my life in the United States than in Senegal. Though I am a U.S. citizen and live here, I do not consider myself "from" here. Still, living in the U.S. has shaped my socialization in many ways. Professionally, I am a professor, a teacher, and a mentor. For the past three years, I've also served as the lead for the Atlantic Fellows for Health Equity program, which brings together people from around the world to share and learn about addressing health disparities.

Obregon: I am a father, husband, son, and friend, roles that deeply shape my personal identity. Culturally, I see myself as Colombian, even though I have lived more years outside Colombia than within it. My identity is enriched by my experiences living and working across Latin America, Africa, and Asia. So, while I am Colombian, my worldview is influenced by these diverse cultural contexts. Professionally, I have worn many _withats, faculty member, consultant, researcher, practitioner, and now manager. Across these roles, I have worked on initiatives aimed at addressing a range of development issues, particularly those connected to communication, development, health, and culture. Despite the diversity of my roles, I primarily identify as a health communicator working in development contexts. A consistent trait across both my cultural and professional identities is that I am a learner, always curious and open to new insights, even on topics I think I already know.

Cultural Dimensions of Health Communication

Airhihenbuwa: In your journey, what has been the role of culture in your communication work?

Obregon: Reflecting on my journey, I began in commercial radio journalism in Colombia before working with the Ministry of Labor's National Apprenticeship Service. In that organization, I engaged in the government's community development initiatives, some of which were inspired by Paulo Freire's pedagogy of liberation and deeply influenced my thinking. We applied Freirean principles in community work, particularly with women-led housing projects in remote and rural areas. This experience helped me see communication as more than media, it became a tool for community engagement and dialogue. As my career progressed, I shifted toward public health, especially in how communication intersects with health and development. In 2014, as the global lead of the Communication for Development area in the Programme Division at UNICEF Headquarters, the Ebola outbreak was pivotal in showing us how cultural understanding and community engagement are essential. Unlike previous epidemics and pandemics, Ebola forced us to listen deeply to communities and consider their oral traditions, cultural practices, and political histories. It challenged the reliance on top-down, biomedical messaging and reinforced the urgency of culture-centered approaches, as emphasized by Sastry and Mohan Dutta (see related references). Community members and networks are often the first responders during crises. For example, Paul Richards' work, in 2016, on Ebola in Sierra Leone, highlights this clearly (see related reference). We saw similar dynamics during Hurricane Katrina in New Orleans. Yet, investments in community structures and networks within health systems remain insufficient. The allocation of resources to preparedness efforts compared to response illustrates this very well. We must recognize and strengthen these preparedness structures to build resilient systems.

Ndiaye: My path also started with media/communication, which I saw as a gateway to development. Eventually, I found my space at the intersection of health, communication, and culture. I came to see that many health communication efforts ignored the cultural identities and norms of communities. As a result, they failed to achieve meaningful outcomes. For me, health communication has been a journey of repetition. We learned lessons during the HIV and Ebola pandemics, but when it's time to develop new interventions, we often revert to ineffective biomedical-only approaches. I've resisted strategies imposed on my culture that dismiss our own ways of making health decisions. Communities communicate about health through culture, whether we recognize it or not.

Building on the Chapter with Current Events

Airhihenbuwa: In what ways would you expand the chapter to reflect more recent events?

Obregon: One important update to this chapter would be to link the chapter's insights to later work, particularly the UNAIDS Communication Framework (see related reference) that identified five key domains, policy, SES, culture, gender, and spirituality, with culture serving as the connecting thread. We should also expand the discussion on literacy. The chapter critiques the approach to literacy when they are disconnected from lived experiences, particularly in the global South. *But we also must rethink literacy as culturally grounded learning*. COVID-19 also revealed the limits of literacy, when even highly educated individuals resisted vaccination, we saw that facts alone are insufficient. While this became salient during the COVID-19 pandemic, we have known for years that highly educated communities, especially in developed countries, have resisted immunization despite the overwhelming evidence regarding their efficacy, safety, and effectiveness.

Ndiaye: I appreciated the chapter's metaphor comparing cultures to eggs or coconuts. Today's cultural landscape is even more dynamic than it was 30 years ago. Systems thinking and human-centered design are more common, but often still carry the same flaws, failing to truly center community voices. *We must stop repeating failed interventions.* During both Ebola and COVID-19, institutions were forced to listen to communities only after all other measures had failed. It shouldn't take a crisis to value community insight.

Airhihenbuwa: At the height of the HIV epidemic, Peter Piot emphasized institutional behavior change, not just individual change. If institutions don't transform, sustainable health improvements won't happen.

Obregon: Human-centered design (HCD), as used today, often co-opts participatory methods rooted in Freirean thinking but lacks their political depth. True participatory work surfaces power dynamics, whereas HCD tends to avoid or bypass them. As technology and social media platforms continue to evolve so rapidly, we should also explore the implications of AI for culture-centered health communication. While AI may bring a lot of positives to health communication, we must ask ourselves to what extent AI may pull health communication practitioners away from culture-centered approaches. Similarly, social media platforms have become forces that can quickly spread misinformation or help address health issues. What role does culture play in the technology and social media ecosystem? These are questions worth exploring from a culture-centered lens.

Ndiaye: Another element worth preserving from the chapter is the idea of cultural agents, like grandparents. In some indigenous communities, certain health-related knowledge is shared only between grandparents and grandchildren, showing the importance of intergenerational communication in traditional healing.

Training the Next Generation

Airhihenbuwa: What should be our focus in training the next generation?

Ndiaye: Today's youth are shaped by hybrid cultures in ways we've never seen. In Butaro, Rwanda, young people act like their peers in Dakar, Lagos, or Washington, D.C. They share global codes through entertainment, yet are not fully Westernized. We must design communication that reflects both their hybrid realities and their historical roots. For instance, storytelling in traditional healing illustrates how health messages can be grounded in shared cultural values. Public vs. private space is also a cultural variable. Conversations about vaccines often involve negotiating which space is appropriate for processing information.

Obregon: Health communication is highly multidisciplinary, which is both a strength and a weakness. Different disciplines bring different biases. Behavioral economics, for example, is increasingly dominating recent health communication strategies, but it often sidelines participatory engagement at the risk of taking us back many years and to a primary focus on individual behavior change. Leaders can shape agendas based on their disciplinary lens, but sometimes at the expense of inclusive dialogue. In addition, efforts to strengthen the positioning of health communication as an established field can benefit from curricular approaches that place culture at the center of training programs, both academic and professional.

Final Thoughts

The conversation traced a shared journey in development and health communication and emphasized the critical role of cultural practices in health communication. Both interviewees expressed frustration with the continued practice of past wrong lessons and stressed the potential of the next generation to center culture in new ways. Success stories, such as using storytelling for mental health and navigating public/private spaces for health messages, showed what's possible when culture is prioritized. They underscored yet again the need to move beyond biomedical dominance and challenge neo-colonial health approaches. The Ebola outbreak and the COVID-19 pandemic served as a wake-up call, proving that culture must be central to public health efforts.

Chapter 3

Developing Culturally Appropriate Health Programs

THEN:

> How we view ourselves, our environment even, is very much dependent on where we stand in relationship to imperialism in its colonial and neo-colonial stages; if we are to do anything about our individual and collective being today, then we have to coldly and consciously look at what imperialism has been doing to us and to our view of ourselves in the universe.
>
> Ngugi Wa Thiong'O, *Decolonizing the Mind*, 1986

The focus on primary health care as the international road map to universal health coverage, commonly referred to as the Alma-Ata Declaration, and subsequently the African ministers of health's introduction of a cost-effective framework for financing primary health care known as the Bamako Initiative, placed the emphasis in global health improvement on primary health care. Public health observers with a commitment to improving health in Southern nations have embraced this focus as realistic and appropriate. There is no single strategy for understanding complex health problems, but an understanding of the complexity of the problems is a prerequisite for the proposal of effective solutions. It is more effective to adapt preventive health programs to fit community needs and cultural contexts than the reverse, hence the need to ensure that public health, communication, and health promotion programs are culturally appropriate. Although several public health, health promotion, and health communication models/frameworks are currently being used in the planning, implementation, and evaluation of preventive health programs, none seem to centralize culture as a critical force in the prevention of disease and the promotion of health.

The training of any person for an occupation requires an understanding of culture as a superstructure, one that preserves remnants of the past within a substructure that is itself undergoing revolutionary transformation. The occupation should also be understood as an instrument through which culture is also transformed. (Freire, 1973). Health beliefs and actions should be examined within the context of culture, history, and politics. In this chapter, I present the PEN-3 model, a conceptual model used in the planning and development of culturally appropriate public health promotion, communication, and education programs (Airhihenbuwa, 1989b, 1990-1991, 1992). To illustrate the model, I discuss its application to child survival interventions in Nigeria. The version of the model presented here is a revision of the original.

Background on Health Education Approaches

Among approaches to health promotion and disease prevention, the self-empowerment method is believed to be more encompassing and more effective than preventive-medical or radical-political approaches. The preventive-medical approach focuses on influencing individual decisions leading to the adoption of positive health behaviors, whereas the radical-political approach focuses on manipulating the social and political environment to tackle ill health at its foundation (Tones, Tilford, & Robinson, 1991, pp.1-16). The preventive-medical approach has a tendency to blame the victim; the radical-political approach can be biased toward the interests and priorities of the health interventionists, even when such interests and priorities are at variance with those of the target community. The self-empowerment approach facilitates choices for individuals within the context of the sociocultural and political environment. This is accomplished through the supplementation of health knowledge acquisition with values clarification and practice skills in decision making through nontraditional teaching methods.

Thus, the self-empowerment method draws on elements of both the preventive-medical and the radical-political approaches (Tones et al., 1991). However, a striking but limiting feature of the self-empowerment approach is the emphasis on the *self*. Such emphasis places the onus of responsibility for health behavior outcome on the individual - a limitation shared with the preventive medical approach. Given this limitation, I use the term *cultural empowerment* here to extend the possibilities of the empowerment approach. Cultural empowerment takes into account how health knowledge, beliefs, and actions are produced and interpreted at both micro (individual, family, and community/grassroots) and macro (national and international power and politics) levels. Thus, the decision-making of individuals and families must be situated within its proper political, historical, and cultural context.

Cultural sensitivity, in health promotion and behavior change programs, refers to the development and adaptation of programs so that they are situated within appropriate cultural frameworks rather than the Western so-called scientific culture within which most health and development programs are planned, implemented, and evaluated. Health results from a process of adaptation. It is the result not of instinct but of an autonomous yet culturally shaped reaction to socially created reality (Illich, 1976).

When present values and practices are not seriously considered in health and development programs, their usefulness within the cultural context of African communities is at best questionable. Thus, to locate culture at the core of health education/promotion programs requires a thorough examination and understanding of the historicity within the cultural and political context of present health beliefs and actions of a people. This is a process of cultural empowerment.

This process of empowering individuals in health education and communication programming is often based on the assumption that individuals, primarily because of their limited economic resources, are powerless. Eurocentrists often consider silence, which makes most Westerners uncomfortable, to indicate voicelessness and weakness. They thus believe that knowledge can be measured using economic/development indices such as income level and fluency in a Western language. Failing to recognize that knowledge born of the Western economic/ developmental praxis carries questionable values and biases that marginalize traditional and local knowledge, Eurocentrists introduced the notion of empowerment in a form of "participation" to legitimate the development concept (Rahnema, 1992). The authoritarian connotation of participation obviously reduces it to a presence of the popular classes in the administration of development programs (Freire, 1993). This silencing of Others through development participation foregrounds the impetus for the construction of a culturally appropriate programmatic framework for health promotion programs in Africa. This process, known as PEN-3, has been employed to guide workshops on child survival in Nigeria as well as workshops on AIDS and diet and exercise among African Americans.

The PEN-3 Model

Any conceptual approach for public health, communication, and health promotion programs should be anchored in a dialogic process that allows members of the targeted culture to address cultural sensitivity and cultural appropriateness in program development. Although I refer to PEN-3 as a model, my intent is not for it to be applied in some prefabricated box or matrix but for it to offer a space within which cultural codes and meanings can be centralized in the development, implementation, and evaluation of health programming.

The PEN-3 model allows the kind of flexibility that encourages intracultural diversity, such that the process should be engaged each time a program is conceived. Health workers should employ a dialogic/polylogue process that ensures affirmation of different cultural expressions in specific locations. Moreover, this method also challenges health and cultural workers to address health issues at the macro (policy, government, societal, and international) level as well as the traditional micro level of health program interventions. The utility of this method, therefore, relates to its amenability to modification and extension of its limits and possibilities, such that the co-creation and acquisition of knowledge in a culture is sensitively and sensibly represented in the project. In addition, this method incorporates existing models/theories and frameworks in health education while drawing on theory and application in cultural studies. Thus, PEN-3 consists of three domains of health, culture, and contexts that are dynamically interrelated and interdependent in shaping behaviors: ***cultural identity*** (referred to originally as health education), ***relationships and expectations*** (referred to originally as educational diagnosis of health behavior), and ***cultural empowerment*** (referred to originally as cultural appropriateness of health behavior).

The PEN-3 model is illustrated in Figure 3.1, which lists the three categories (according to the acronym PEN) within each of the three domains. The first domain of the PEN-3 model is cultural identity, the three categories of which are person, extended family, and neighborhood.

Person. Cultural Identity is central to how we understand the health of all. To this end, individuals should be engaged to have their voices heard before making any health decision that affects them, their families, and their communities.

Extended family. Cultural Identity is central to decisions that affect not only the immediate, nuclear family but also extended kin. Such a focus on the extended family should also consider family lineage (e.g., patrilinear or matrilinear). However, when a program is designed to target a particular member of the family (e.g., the mother), the individual should become the focus of the study and must be so recognized. Such recognition must be noted within the context of the individual's environment.

Neighborhood. Cultural Identity is central to promoting health and preventing disease in neighborhoods and communities. Involvement of community members and their leaders becomes critical in the provision of culturally appropriate health programs. In fact, because community leadership often defines community boundaries, it is critical for leaders to define what constitutes their community or neighborhood at the beginning of a project.

Figure 3.1: PEN-3

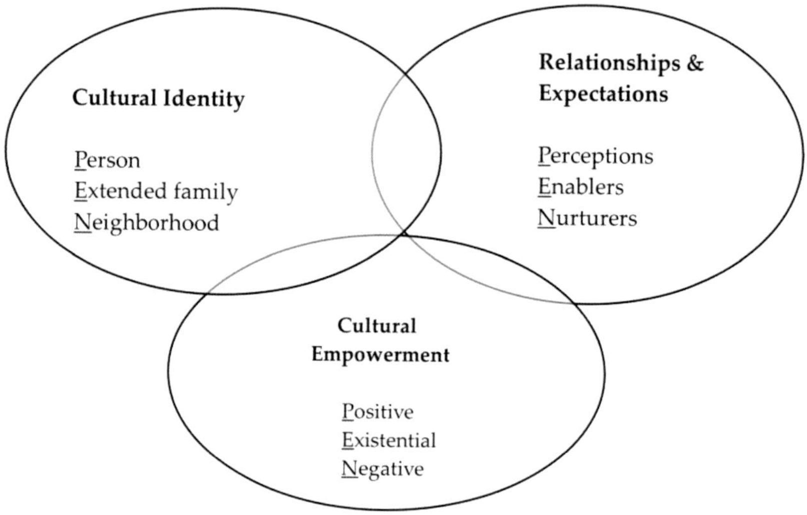

The second dimension of PEN-3 is the relationships and expectations of one's role in the family and community. Within this domain, the categories of perception and enablers have been used by researchers to attempt to determine the factors that influence individual, family, and/or community health actions. Some of the models or frameworks that have been used in understanding and predicting health-related behaviors are the health belief model (Rosenstock, 1974), Fishbein and Ajzen's (1975) theory of reasoned action, and the PRECEDE framework (Mullen, Hersey, & Iverson, 1987). Influenced by Kurt Lewin's (1947) "life space" notion, the health belief model deals with individuals' perceptions of their susceptibility to disease and of the severity of their diseases as predictors of their health actions. Fishbein and Ajzen's theory of reasoned action postulates that behavioral intention is a function of attitude toward performance of an impending behavior reinforced by feedback from significant others. The PRECEDE-PROCEED framework (Green & Kreuter, 1991) deals with how to identify, change/modify, and evaluate which health-related and non-health-related behaviors are most important and changeable, considering personal, family, community, and environmental factors.

This domain of PEN-3 has evolved from the confluence of the three aforementioned models. However, it is important to note that culture has no central role in these earlier models. PEN-3, therefore, extends the possibilities advanced in previous models and frameworks by placing culture at the core of public health, health promotion, and disease prevention programs. The categories in the second dimension of the PEN-3 approach are perceptions, enablers, and nurturers.

Perceptions. Perceptions comprise the knowledge, attitudes, values, and beliefs, within a cultural context, that may facilitate or hinder personal, family, and community motivation to change. For example, some Nigerian mothers believe that a healthy child does not need to be protected against illness, and this may affect immunization programs, because preventive injections have always been considered treatment. Or, for instance, if there is a cultural belief that consuming sweet foods causes diarrhea (a belief held by some Edos, Yorubas, and Igbos of Nigeria), it will be a serious challenge to promote the use of homemade oral rehydration solutions, which contain sugar, as therapy for diarrhea. Existing perceptions can lead to the need to resolve conflicts that might arise in people's minds, because to them it might seem as though the causative agent of a disease is also its cure. For example, when African Americans have answered yes to the question "Can someone get AIDS from donating blood?" some researchers have misinterpreted this to mean they have poor AIDS knowledge. In fact, this response sometimes indicates a strong negative distrust of White health care providers, reflecting a belief that they may intentionally infect Blacks with the AIDS virus - a perception that is a legacy of the US Public Health Service syphilis experiments that were conducted in Tuskegee, which has become a legacy of medical racism in general. In regard to differences in perception of body weight between African Americans and Whites, several researchers have reported that being overweight is not necessarily associated with negative body image for many African Americans (e.g., Desmond, Price, Hallinan, & Smith, 1989; Kumanyika, Wilson, & Guilford-Davenport, 1993). African Americans who are heavy or above normal weight are likely to perceive themselves as having a normal body weight than their White counterparts. In fact, in one study, 40% of African American women who were classified as overweight considered their figures attractive or very attractive. However, such perceptions about body image should not compromise the seriousness of obesity as a predisposing factor to chronic degenerative conditions such as type II diabetes and heart disease.

Enablers. Enablers are cultural, societal, systematic, or structural influences or forces that may enhance or be barriers to change, such as the availability of resources, accessibility, referrals, employers, government officials, skills, and types of services (e.g., traditional medicine). At a child survival workshop in Nigeria, several mothers cited being asked to pay for the treatment of abscesses (a side effect of vaccination) as a major reason for not taking their children for immunization through the Expanded Program on Immunization (EPI), even though they know the injections are free. Paulo Freire discovered that mothers' reluctance and/or refusal to give eggs to their children started when colonial settlers told the indigenes that eggs were bad for them (the indigenes), so that eggs would be sold cheaply (because they were of little use to those who produced them) to the colonizers (in Freire & Faundez, 1989). Finally, opportunity costs are always an important factor to be considered in the planning and implementation of health intervention programs for African American communities.

Nurturers. Another important element is the degree to which health beliefs, attitudes, and actions are influenced and mediated, or nurtured, by extended family, kin, friends, peers, and the community. For example, the fact that older siblings who were never immunized are in good health tends to suggest to some grandparents that EPI (Expanded Program on Immunization) and other modern preventive actions against childhood diseases are unwarranted for their younger grandchildren. The concept of nurturers emphasizes the importance of significantly increasing the number of African Americans in the health professions who understand and respect African American culture and communities. It is also important to promote an understanding of cultural beliefs and practices among non-African Americans. For example, because of the disproportionately high level of cardiovascular disease in the African American population, special emphasis has been placed on eating practices and weight control. Because food is a cultural symbol and eating is a symbolic act through which people communicate, perpetuate, and develop their knowledge and attitudes toward life, an understanding of cultural influences on eating habits is essential for the health educator who wants to provide realistic educational interventions designed to modify dietary practices (Kaufman-Kurzrock, 1989).

The third and most critical domain of the PEN-3 model is cultural empowerment. This domain is pivotal to the development of a culturally sensitive health and communication program. This domain situates culture in dynamic and interacting forces that manifest themselves in individual, family, and community behavior. Each of these three domains can relate to perceptions, enablers, and nurturers within their historical and cultural contexts. This final domain consists of the categories of positive, existential, and negative behaviors.

Positive behaviors. These are behaviors that are based on health beliefs and actions that are known to be beneficial and must be encouraged. These behaviors are critical in the empowerment of persons, extended families, and neighborhoods. *Affirmation of these behaviors is critical to program success and sustainability, particularly because they are examples of these cultures' contributions to the global production of knowledge and meaning*. Examples include the promotion of such traditional practices as breastfeeding and the consuming green vegetables. There is a tendency on the part of upwardly mobile African American professionals to disengage slowly from eating green vegetables, as was done traditionally, because such foods are not believed to be associated with progress and affluence.

Existential behaviors. Existential behaviors comprise those cultural beliefs, practices, and/or behaviors that are indigenous to a group and have no harmful health consequences, and thus need not be targeted for change and should not be blamed for program failure simply because they are ill understood. An example is the use of palm oil and indigo as a soothing lotion for a child with measles. Another example is the placing of an amulet around a child's neck to ward off evil spirits. In fact, some physicians have used this practice with their pediatric patients, telling them that only the physicians may remove the amulets. This helps to guarantee that patients will return for follow-up visits.

Public health and communication scholars and practitioners should address *what is* and not *what ought to be*. They should refrain from moralizing over behaviors that are unfamiliar to them and that they do not understand. The programmatic thrust of public health and communication should be to address *what is* in terms of matching intervention with current health practices, such as sexual activities among teenagers, rather than *what ought to be*, such as abstinence. Understanding these existential beliefs is where African American theoreticians have made significant contributions. For example, these researchers link African American lifestyles, at least in part, with African values to produce a holistic worldview, as opposed to an abstract construction of personality assessment that sees the individual as pathological.

Negative behaviors. Negative behaviors are based on health beliefs and actions that are known to be harmful to health: Health providers must therefore examine and understand them within their cultural, historical, and political contexts before attempting to change them. Examples of negative behaviors include the withholding of fluid from a victim of diarrhea and unprotected sexual intercourse.

In PEN-3, the *Es - extended family, enablers, and existential behaviors - are the most powerful influences on and for cultural production.* The enablers speak to power, politics, and history; the existential speaks to affirmation of humanity and cultural empowerment; and extended family speaks to the vitality of sustained positive traditions and influence, as well as a major contribution to global production of knowledge, meaning, and interpretation. *The dynamic interrelatedness of these three levels must be balanced to demonstrate the degree to which politics, policy, power, and culture shape and are being shaped by individuals and the family.*

Health, communication, and education programs involve health beliefs and behaviors. These programs must reflect the cultural perspectives of the people for whom they are designed. Researchers and practitioners should focus on both positive (cultural empowerment process) and negative behaviors in a health program. Very often, too much attention is focused on negative behaviors, with few or no rewards offered for positive behaviors. In some instances, interventionists arrogantly blame the failure to change negative behaviors on the presence of existential behaviors.

The process of culturalizing health knowledge, attitudes, and practices must not assume that people are powerless or ignorant. The process affirms diversity in the way people construct their individual and collective realities within the possibilities of their locations. What is positive or negative cannot be based on a universal notion promoted in economic development. In fact, the process challenges the shortcomings of empowerment as advanced in the economic/development paradigm. Rahnema (1992) illustrates these shortcomings in the following:

> When A considers it essential for B to be empowered, A assumes not only that B has no power, or does not have the right kind of power, but also that A has the secret formula of a power to which B has to be initiated. In the current *participatory ideology*, this formula is, in fact, nothing but a revised version of state power, or what could be called fear-power. The crux of the matter is that populations actually subjected to this fear-power are not at all powerless. (p.123; emphasis added)

Implementation of Child Survival Programs

The PEN-3 model was operationalized at the African Regional Child Survival Workshop in Nigeria, June-July 1990, and subsequently at the training of trainers workshop for Africare and the Imo (Nigeria) State Ministry of Health. A total of 20 participants from 10 different African countries representing 10 nongovernmental organizations (NGOs) with child survival projects were assigned to four intervention groups: oral rehydration therapy (ORT), EPI, nutrition, and high-risk birth. Based on their child survival field experiences, each group developed a list of reported positive, existential, and negative health beliefs related to their assigned interventions. These health beliefs reflected the perceptions, enablers, and nurturers of members of the communities for whom the child survival projects were designed. With the information generated on positive, existential, and negative health beliefs, each intervention group developed a list of interview questions (according to perceptions, enablers, and nurturers) for one of four preselected segments of the community. The four segments of the community that were interviewed were mothers, village health workers, traditional leaders, and local government representatives. Information about child survival interventions was obtained from the community on perceptions (beliefs related to knowledge, attitudes, and practices), enablers (culture, structure, skills, and resources necessary for health actions), and nurturers (family, kin, and friend reinforcement for health beliefs and practices). The participants then classified the items into positive, existential, and negative health beliefs and practices to delineate appropriately the focus for health promotion and disease prevention in the community.

At the end of the first workshop, a second was held with the staff of the Ministry of Health, who provide training for the village health workers in the area. At this second workshop, the information generated at the first was used to classify health beliefs into two categories. Listed below are the beliefs that were identified under the domain of cultural identity. Each belief/practice is labeled either T, for a long-term health belief that is deeply rooted in the tradition and culture, or R, for a recent and short-term health belief that may or may not become part of long-term tradition.

Positive: Cultural Empowerment

1. The idea of taking fluids during illness is acceptable. T
2. The community noticed a decline in diarrhea morbidity/mortality with ORT usage. R
3. Community leaders are willing and able to take the lead as change agents. T
4. The giving of plantain porridge to children who have diarrhea is acceptable. T
5. The giving of pap and/or coconut juice to children who have diarrhea is acceptable. T
6. Sexual abstinence during pregnancy reduces the incidence of pelvic inflammatory disease. T

Existential: No Threat to Health

1. Beads around a child's wrist and/or ankle will ward off evil spirits. T
2. Postpartum sexual abstinence prevents semen from mixing with breast milk. T
3. Palm oil and indigo serve as a good soothing lotion for measles. T
4. Families should have a lot of children because of high child mortality rates. R
5. Women should have all the children that God gives them. T

Negative: Threat to Health

1. Male dominance inhibits necessary female participation. T/R

2. Feeding a child certain foods, such as eggs and meat, causes the child to steal. T

3. Eating sugar and other sweet foods causes diarrhea. T

4. Medicine is needed for diarrhea, and ORT is not medicine. R

5. Babies with diarrhea must not be breastfed. T

6. A healthy child does not need health care; therefore, immunization is unnecessary. T

7. Immunization may cause disability and/or death in a child. R

8. Because older, living, healthy siblings were not immunized, there is no reason to immunize infants. R

9. Contraceptives and tetanus toxoid cause sterility. R

10. A pregnant woman's eating eggs, meat, or chicken causes her baby to be too big to deliver normally. T

11. Taking fluids during diarrhea will prolong diarrhea and/or result in the development of worms. T

The health workers then conducted a workshop with the village health workers to discuss these health beliefs, particularly those that are rooted in tradition and culture. It should be noted that the above dichotomy does not represent a static classification. This classification was provided by health workers who train the village health workers. What is traditional or recent may vary from one location to another.

Application of the Model

In the development of programs that fit in with a community's existing beliefs and practices, the PEN-3 model can be utilized, as illustrated by the steps taken in the workshops described above. In the first phase, the program planners must determine whether the emphasis of the program will be on the person, the extended family, or the neighborhood (cultural empowerment), realizing that these are not mutually exclusive categories. In the second phase, the interventionists should explore (through interviews and/or surveys) the beliefs and practices related to perceptions, enablers, and nurturers (relationships and expectations). Such examinations will relate to a particular health issue in different segments of the family or community. On the basis of the information generated, in the third phase, the interventionists should categorize the different beliefs and practices found into positive, existential, and negative beliefs (cultural identity). Finally, with the assistance and guidance of a community facilitator such as a health coach, the interventionists should classify all the health beliefs into two groups: those that are historically rooted in the cultural patterns and lifestyle of the target community, and those that are newly formulated and have only superficial ties with the cultural patterns and lifestyle of the target community.

Discussion

The implementation of interventions, consistent with PEN-3, should be based on whether health beliefs and behaviors are long-term and historically rooted in the tradition and culture or more recent, short-term beliefs. The reinforcement or changing of long-term cultural beliefs should be addressed through health education in the home (home visits) and/or through one-to-one contacts in the community, whereas more recent, non-traditionally entrenched health beliefs could be addressed through traditional media - posters, flyers, radio and television messages, and so on (Airhihenbuwa, 1992; Fuglesang, 1973) or using different social media platforms. It should be noted, however, that although home visits may also be appropriate for changing non-entrenched health beliefs, mass media have not proved effective for changing negative health beliefs that are historically rooted in cultural patterns and lifestyles. Researchers have shown that mass media channels are most effective for increasing knowledge, reinforcing previously held attitudes, and changing behaviors that were recently established or predisposed to change, as opposed to those that are tied to cultural values or are contrary to the attitudes and values expressed in the mass media (Griffiths & Knutson,1960). In child survival programs, despite the difficulty in organizing an outreach, face-to-face communication channels were found to be most effective in educating mothers about the use of oral rehydration therapy for persons with diarrhea (Hornik, 1988).

The health promotion and communication specialists must understand the rationale behind stated beliefs and practices. To emphasize this point, the Ministry of Health trainers at the workshop discussed above were asked to supervise their village health workers in role plays on health beliefs. This was necessary for them to be able to make appropriate classifications and to select appropriate health education strategies. Moreover, this exercise provided an important demonstration of the ubiquitous nature of some of these beliefs relative to the three domains of positive, existential, and negative, and how a given belief may be functional in more than one category, depending on the objective of the health program. For example, when classifying beliefs and practices into positive, existential, and negative beliefs, "Families should have a lot of children because of high child mortality rates" could be classified as a negative belief. However, the health workers in this case classified it as existential, because this belief, which is logical, is a reality for the women living in this community. On the other hand, it could become a positive belief in a vaccination program designed to motivate individuals and families to have fewer children. In another example, the belief that postpartum sexual abstinence prevents semen from mixing with breast milk can be positive in terms of child spacing and allowing a woman ample time to recover following the strain of childbirth. The classification of "immunization as a cause of death" is an example of a recent, non-culturally entrenched belief resulting from actual experience. This belief was established when some children who had been immunized through EPI later died, after their mothers were told that immunization would prevent their children's deaths. Only face-to-face education has been effective in convincing mothers that immunization may prevent a child from dying from some diseases and that additional preventive measures must be taken to protect children against other illnesses, such as diarrhea and malaria.

Regarding political and institutional factors, another example is helpful. Some health workers had observed that women from certain areas were not taking their children to be immunized. Upon inquiry by an expert trusted by the women, it was discovered that there were cases of children who developed side effects, such as abscesses, from immunization. In addition, the women were asked to pay for treatment of this resultant condition, even though EPI services are free. The health workers recommended to the authorities at the Ministry of Health that they evaluate and try to eliminate any adverse consequences of immunization, and that the ministry should provide treatment free of charge in those cases in which a problem does develop.

When dealing with oral traditions, the focus should not be limited to "how to transform the learner," as is often the case; rather, attention should also be paid to whether the interventionist has the requisite skill to engage and share knowledge in a culturally appropriate manner. *It is important not only to understand the storyteller; it is equally important, if not more so, to understand the dynamics of the story listener.* Oral tradition generally is not the heritage solely of the spoken or sung word; it is also the heritage of the ear (Faseke, 1990). Stated differently, people in the oral traditional cultures of several African countries are accustomed to learning by what they hear. Learning by what they see is important to the extent that it is congruent with what they hear and who produces that information. The implication of this pattern of knowledge acquisition for the teacher must be understood and appropriately employed. In other words, if people in an oral traditional culture learn more by listening, the teacher (health educator) should spend more time talking, discussing, and sharing insights than showing pictures or using other audiovisual aids. If talking and sharing ideas constitute the primary mode of learning, health providers (particularly those from other countries) must have adequate competence in oral communication to be able to impart knowledge effectively to individuals, families, and the community.

Lessons From HIV/AIDS Prevention

In response to the need for a culturally appropriate health intervention framework, the PEN-3 method was used to guide the development of an HIV/AIDS education program so as to ensure that cultural beliefs and experiences were considered in exploring and promoting behavior change. The involvement of community members is the key to an adequate assessment of culturally relevant health beliefs and practices and to the planning of appropriate interventions. Jaccard, Turrisi, and Wan (1990) propose that after the high-risk activities of a target population have been identified, two strategies should be considered in attempting to change these behaviors. The first is environmental transformation, which involves altering or improving structural features in the environment that will provide opportunities for the adoption of alternate behaviors. Examples of this strategy include the provision of clean needles to reduce the frequency of needle sharing among intravenous drug users and the provision of condoms to reduce the frequency of unprotected sexual intercourse.

The second strategy is persuasive communication, or the deliberate influencing and modifying of individual beliefs, attitudes, and/ or decisions through exposure to information. Source expertise is a critical factor in the use of persuasive communication in AIDS education programs designed for African American communities. Practitioners and researchers should include underrepresented minority members, because these individuals are more knowledgeable than others about the behaviors and values of their communities (Peterson & Bakerman, 1989).

Language, both verbal and nonverbal, is a critical tool of persuasive communication. This must be understood by those attempting to select appropriate interventions for racial or ethnic groups. The reinforcement or changing of cultural beliefs should be attempted within the context of the culture's lexicon.

A form of communication prevalent among many African Americans is African American English (AAE), a well-formed and valid linguistic system that encompasses the whole range of language forms used by African Americans throughout the United States (McNair-Knox, 1991). A variation of AAE is African American Vernacular English (AAVE), more commonly called Black Vernacular English or Ebonics, which is associated with the speech of low-income African Americans, particularly young people. The cultural rationale for understanding AAVE is that its use among teens appears to function as an important symbol of peer group solidarity and as a demonstration of pride in African heritage. In Nigeria, the use of Naija language (commonly referred to as pidgin or broken English) is an example of understanding and engaging with a language that speaks to the heart of the population. Naija language is at the center of the global presence and dominance of Afrobeat music and Nollywood movies from Nigeria. Culturally embodied language is a window to underlying messages that connect one's identity to issues around behavioral norms, and collection reactions to environmental conditions. Efforts to tap into this expression may create a relatively positive and nonthreatening context for communicating health messages. Therefore, HIV/AIDS prevention messages must be developed and communicated in a manner that ensures their reception by the members of the groups at greatest risk.

Conclusion

Several cultural factors can promote or hinder the success of health education programs in the global south countries. The future of public health interventions, health promotion, and communication lies in the ability to centralize these cultural factors within their proper historical and political contexts. For health interventionists, particularly in countries of Africa, Latin America, and Asia as well as among ethnic minority populations in industrialized nations, practitioners and researchers must employ culturally sensitive methods to examine varied health behaviors in terms of positive/beneficial beliefs that must be encouraged, existential/cultural beliefs and practices that do not threaten health, and negative/harmful health practices that should be changed.

In the chapters that follow, I discuss the politics of representation within the context of population subgroups and traditional healing modalities. Examples of the PEN-3 method are presented within the context of each chapter. The examples are meant to generate more discussion, so that cultural domains of health can be assessed from positive, existential, and negative perspectives rather than from the sole perspective of negativity. Such negativity has led to the almost automatic coupling of the concept of cultural difference with that of barriers. The PEN-3 examples, therefore, are designed to transform the notion of *cultural barriers* to *cultural domains*, wherein strengths are acknowledged, and barriers are understood as one unfortunate outcome better understood within their contexts.

NOW:

My Conversation with Juliet I. Iwelunmor, Ucheoma C. Nwaozuru

Cultural and Professional Identities

Airhihenbuwa: See my intro in chapter one

Iwelunmor: I am a mother, daughter, wife, sister, friend, and sibling. It's hard to pin down where one stands these days because so much is shifting in so many directions. But if I had to define who I am, I would say I'm a passerby in this world, destined to tell stories about how we sustain our well-being through the connections we build with family and community. Professionally, I'm a professor of medicine at Washington University School of Medicine and the founder of the LIGHT Institute at Washington University in St. Louis, where we focus on sustaining evidence-based health interventions in low-resource settings.

Nwaozuru: I see myself as a friend, sister, daughter, and neighbor, depending on who is around me. Culturally, I identify as an Igbo Nigerian. That identity is central to me, especially having lived in the U.S. for 15 years. It's difficult for me to fully assume an American identity or even to see myself as Black, as that label usually only comes up in professional spaces. So culturally, I identify as a woman who is Igbo and Nigerian. Professionally, I'm a researcher interested in the intersection of technology, entrepreneurship, social innovation, and health. I'm deeply focused on reflecting the true voices and strengths of communities in helping them live healthy lives. That orientation is tied to my cultural background, where communal growth and learning are emphasized.

The Continuing Relevance of the PEN-3 Model Today

Airhihenbuwa: PEN-3 was introduced over 35 years ago, before it became a chapter in *Health and Culture*. Iwelunmor, you conducted the first systematic review of the model in 2014, and Nwaozuru, you completed the most recent review in the 2022 book

Health, Culture and Place. The question for our conversation is: Is this chapter on PEN-3 still relevant today?

Iwelunmor: I think now more than ever, it remains deeply relevant. I'd like to believe that when you created it, you may not have anticipated it would become such an ambitious tool, one that challenges people to move beyond single lenses. The chapter opens with Achebe's quote: "Where one thing stands, another will stand beside it." That duality captures what PEN-3 stands for. Even in the chaos of today's academic environment, we still find clarity, where chaos exists, clarity stands beside it. *PEN-3 reminds us that the challenges and hurdles in health are not isolated; the solutions, particularly the cultural ones, are often wrapped within those hurdles*. That's the beauty, the genius, and the ambition of PEN-3: it remains applicable to any health issue, any context.

When we say, "public health," we often emphasize the "health" and forget the "public." PEN-3 redirects our focus to the public, prompting us to consider not only the challenges but also the nurturing aspects within communities, perceptions, relationships, and resources. The model compels us to ask whether these aspects are enabling or hindering, and how they shape our interventions. It trains us to see both the hurdles and the possibilities wrapped around them.

Airhihenbuwa: As I revisited the chapter, I noted how the names of the domains have evolved. The Cultural Empowerment domain was originally "health education"; Relationship and Expectations was "educational diagnosis of behavior"; and Cultural Identity was "cultural appropriateness of health behavior." These shifts illustrate how far we've come in disentangling public health from strictly clinical and medical paradigms. Back then, programs began with community diagnosis and later became community assessment, especially in schools of public health like UNC-Chapel Hill. These name changes also reflect the constraints of earlier professional norms, how the language of the book in 1995 was shaped by the field of health education and health promotion. But systematic reviews, like yours, Iwelunmor, in 2014 and Nwaozuru's in 2022, show PEN-3's broader relevance today. The lesson remains: focus not only on the problem but on the promise. Nwaozuru, since you led the most recent systematic review, what has your journey with PEN-3 been like? Do you see it as still relevant?

Nwaozuru: Absolutely, PEN-3 remains very relevant. What makes it unique is how it highlights cultural elements that are often overlooked. Human beings tend to categorize things as positive or negative, it's easier for our brain to make sense of it that way. But PEN-3 invites us to look beyond that binary and pay attention to unique characteristics that really matter within a context. It promotes a strengths-based approach, which we are increasingly advocating for today, rather than a deficit model. Looking ahead, I think the Cultural Identity domain deserves renewed attention, especially as our understanding of identities evolve. The concept of family, for example, may be different for younger generations. Individuals may see their social or online spaces as integral to their identities or as an important component of who they consider to be family. So, there's room to expand the model to reflect these shifts. *PEN-3 is evergreen because it prioritizes the importance of community and recognizes its strengths, especially through the existential domain, which helps us uncover and understand what we often overlook.* It's a model that evolves with the times, and that's why it remains so powerful.

The Role of PEN-3 in Implementation Science and Community Engagement

Airhihenbuwa: You (Nwaozuru) talked about the current moment we're in and how social media shapes people's decisions. You're in a department focused on implementation science. In this next part of our conversation, let's talk about culture in the work we do. You introduced yourself earlier as an Igbo woman living in the U.S., which you described as central to your identity. You also mentioned that younger generations may not relate to the idea of extended family in the same way, but feel connected through social or digital spaces. So, within the context of implementation science, how are you navigating culture in your work?

Nwaozuru: In implementation science, which is about closing the gap between research and real-world practice, PEN-3 has helped me think more intentionally about the people we engage. Stakeholder engagement, especially with communities of interest, is essential. To implement anything in the real world, it must be grounded in the community's knowledge and capabilities. PEN-3 enables that. It also brings a health equity lens to implementation science by focusing on community strengths. We talk a lot about "intervention fit" or the "acceptability" of an intervention, but that fit isn't possible unless you understand the unique strengths and values of the individuals or the setting you're working with.

PEN-3 also reminds us that cultural identity matters. People don't exist in isolation, they carry values, histories, and identities that remain meaningful regardless of their environment. We can't just push out an evidence-based intervention and expect it to work without involving the very people it's meant to serve. So, PEN-3 grounds my work in community engagement, ensuring that the solutions are meaningful and sustainable, because they emerge from the lived realities and capabilities of the people themselves.

Sustainability and Global Health Implementations

Airhihenbuwa: Iwelunmor, you've been a catalyst in reimagining what implementation science should be. You led the development of the PLAN model, which is not just about another framework but really about culture. You've spoken about the tendency in public health to emphasize *health* while often neglecting the *public*. You've challenged us to re-inscribe "public" meaningfully into our work. Could you discuss two key aspects: first, the evolution of PLAN as a framework for integrating sustainability into our work; and second, how PEN-3 remains relevant today, particularly in light of its publication and inclusion. The chapter focused on child survival and HIV. Today, youth engagement has become central. What new examples would you suggest for illuminating PEN-3's future application?

Iwelunmor: Even though I led it, developing PLAN was truly a team effort, Nwaozuru was part of that team. The model feels intuitive now: that people shouldn't just do work for the sake of it, but for its long-term benefit. Yet, we found in our research that many investigators say they want their work to be sustainable, but when asked *how*, most have no plan. Literally, no PLAN. As we stated in our paper, many assumed someone else would take over the work after funding ended. This raises a fundamental question: *Why are we doing this work in the first place? Is it just for another publication?* As Toni Morrison once said, we should do work that is not only beautiful and powerful but also work. We don't need another strategy paper that ends up sitting in a journal with no real-world impact, papers that do not work or connect to real-world issues. People who need this work often aren't even considered in the sustainability plan.

So, PLAN begins with P, *People*. Whether you're working with policymakers or youth, their voices matter just as much as those of the so-called experts. We've been intentional about that, especially in our work with young people. What's the point of doing HIV work "for" them if they're not co-designing it? But we also know youth can't scale programs alone. You need policymakers, too. Just this past summer, our STAR Scholars program, a program, dedicated to stimulating interests in HIV research among young people, designed a brilliant project focused on using vending machines for HIV self-testing, with the goal of placing them around the St. Louis area. They pitched the idea to the city health department's HIV division, which, as it turned out, had been thinking about similar issues. That's the power of connection. When you bring the right people together, ideas align in ways that foster impact.

The next piece is L, *Learning*. Once there's evidence, you must take time to learn from it. Even if your approach is innovative, and we value innovation, learning requires that you take a step back and see what works or doesn't work in ways that foster pivotal questions on how to make the ideas work. We learn knowing that so many have paved the way in addressing similar problems. Our job is to continue where they left off, contributing solutions that open doors. Then comes A, *Adaptation*. Sustainability requires adaptation. As PEN-3 teaches us, change is not only inevitable, it's necessary. Most of us grew up without cell phones; now our children wear smartwatches. Our science must adapt just as we do. Your methods, your strategies, your frameworks, everything should be open to change. Finally, N, *Nurturing*. This is about sustaining what has been built: the people, the learning, the changes. You bring values to the table, but so does everyone else. Sustainability is about nurturing those contributions, so the work lives on. That's PLAN: *People, Learning, Adaptation, and Nurturing*, not just doing work for its own sake but ensuring it remains impactful long after you've stepped away.

Now, to your second point, relevance. When the PEN-3 chapter was written, child survival and HIV were major global concerns. The chapter also touched on the uncertainty around HIV/AIDS. Today, we've lived through the COVID-19 pandemic, a once-in-a-generation experience. We now know what it means to wear a mask, to homeschool children, to witness public health succeed in some areas and fall short in others. We saw vaccines that worked but weren't trusted, leading to a crisis of misinformation. Yet, people have long studied how information travels, channels, audiences, and credibility. But during the pandemic, those experts were often nowhere to be found. PEN-3 can guide us to reflect on this. Because another pandemic will come, we don't know when, but it will, and we must be ready.

This reflection shouldn't be for the sake of "experts" alone. Child survival wasn't just about the child being sick; it was about securing a future. The next generation matters. Unfortunately, we only tend to engage children when they are ill or silent. We need to rethink that. We need to imagine not just child *survival* but child *resilience*, ensuring children are not only alive, but thriving, so that they remain central to public health efforts today, not later. And I'll also add, cancer is another area where PEN-3 remains relevant, especially cancers we can eliminate, like cervical cancer. These issues affect people across geographical spaces. The lessons learned in Nigeria can inform strategies in St. Louis. If we don't consider the cost of learning and adaptation, then what's the point? These health innovations won't go anywhere. So yes, PEN-3 can help us focus on people, learning, adaptation, and nurturing, and bring more people into the conversation beyond just the "experts."

Future Direction on PEN-3 Cultural Model

Airhihenbuwa: What are some final thoughts about the future application of the PEN-3 model?

Nwaozuru: One area I would suggest exploring is how to develop quantitative measures for the model's domains. I think introducing quantitative components could expand the utilization of PEN-3. While the model has always been strong qualitatively, having a quantitative framework could help make it more accessible to a wider range of scholars and practitioners who rely on metrics in their work. Another area would be considering developing a web tool to guide the application of PEN-3 in research and other projects. I would also love to see the principles of PEN-3 play out in our personal lives, beyond our research, where it shapes our interactions with people and our communities, centered on their strengths and not just the negatives.

Airhihenbuwa: I appreciate that suggestion. The idea of developing quantitative measures for PEN-3 has come up before. My stance has always been intentional: to leave it open primarily for qualitative exploration. One reason is the prevailing tension between qualitative and quantitative approaches, where qualitative methods are often treated as subordinate to quantitative ones. I, along with others, believe that qualitative research holds its own independent space and merit. It doesn't need validation through numbers to be credible or valuable. That said, if others find ways to use PEN-3 quantitatively, I welcome that. But I will continue to emphasize and protect its qualitative foundation.

Iwelunmor: I agree completely. I don't believe PEN-3 needs to be quantified to achieve its purpose. In fact, the essence of the model is rooted in storytelling. PEN-3 has been at the forefront of telling a deeper story about culture and health in ways that rip the veil open to what is good, what is unique, and the hurdles to address when it comes to the health of a people. It's about capturing the lived experiences and perspectives of people, something that quantitative tools often overlook. *The art of storytelling is exactly what we need when working at the intersection of culture and health.* PEN-3 is powerful because it gives voice to the population in ways that are deeply contextual, deeply nuanced, and profoundly human.

Final Thoughts

In this conversation, we reflected on the continued relevance and evolution of the PEN-3 model. We discussed its original application to child survival and HIV, and how its principles apply today to broader public health concerns such as youth engagement, pandemic preparedness, and cancer prevention. Together, we reaffirmed that PEN-3 remains an evergreen model, one that urges us to look beyond problems to the promises embedded within communities, and to reimagine public health in ways that are sustainable, inclusive, and culturally grounded.

Chapter 4

Health, Healing, and Medicine as Cultural Constructs

THEN:

> To distinguish the doctor's professional exercise of white magic from his function as an engineer (and to spare him the charge of being a quack), the term "placebo" was created. Whenever a sugar pill works because it is given by the doctor, the sugar pill acts as a placebo. A placebo (Latin for "I will please") pleases not only the patient but the administering physician as well.
>
> *Ivan Illich*, Medical Nemesis, 1976

Traditional healing is perhaps the only health system that is accessible to everyone in Africa. Some 80% of Africans use traditional healing methods (Bannerman, Burton, & Wen-Chieh, 1983). Traditional healing has been sustained over the years partly because it is based on cultural values and norms of the people and partly because it is available, acceptable, and affordable.

Africans' use of traditional remedies to prevent, treat, and cure illness dates back several centuries. In examining health services in Africa, as well as in other parts of the world, health educators and designers of health promotion programs must consider the cultural framework carefully to understand how indigenous peoples view sickness, disease, and appropriate treatment methods (Airhihenbuwa, 1990-1991; Harvey, 1988).

Researchers who study health practices and beliefs are now cognizant of the fact that patients and clients who seek prevention or cure for illness or disease do so in a variety of ways, and that prevention and cure are sought from a variety of sources (Dennis, 1985). Moreover, it is now well understood that the sources of prevention and cure of problems are determined to a great extent by the clients' sociocultural and religious backgrounds (Airhihenbuwa, 1987; Holzer, 1973). Because Africa's cultural evolution has often been misrepresented, it is no surprise that its healing modalities have been victims of allopathic hegemony. In Africa, the harsh experiences and upheavals of the slave trade, colonialism, and neocolonialism precluded the pattern of development experienced in the West. Similarly, the evolution of traditional medicine in African countries is different from that of countries that were not colonized, such as China.

In all forms of traditional healing, religion and shared cultural values and beliefs are at the core of preventive and curative health practices. Religion, magic, and superstition, and their resulting practices (e.g., traditional medicine) are all based on rationality. Such rationality is best understood in its traditional (emic) context rather than through a Western (etic) paradigm, hence the popular utilization of traditional medicine in the global south. An etic approach is one that focuses on universal traits regardless of culture, whereas an emic approach focuses on cultural differences (Pike, 1954, cited in Pedersen, Draguns, Conner, & Trimble, 1981; see also Kegley & Saviers, 1983). However, it is useful for public health professionals and health educators to explore the possibilities offered by both systems of medicine, so that Africans can utilize the most effective health care services for different conditions and under differing circumstances.

Reappraisal of Traditional Health Care

It is a commonly and easily observed fact that even the most "detribalized" and "modernized" Christians, scholars, scientists, and entrepreneurs among the African bourgeoisie today still consult African divinities, diviners, and healers when their health or other affairs are in serious trouble. Many have been known to sneak away from their church pews, discard their three-piece suits, steal away by night to some healer in his displaced shrine, and carry out all manner of ritual sacrifices when these are demanded. In fact, even among those with Ph.D.s, D.Sc.s, LL.D.s, and other assorted strings of Western bourgeois academic degrees, the going attitude is still that Western medicines and the Western Christian God are fine in their place, but when things get tough, one runs back to one's roots and ancestral ways (Chinweizu, Jemie, & Madubuike, 1983, p.21).

The existence or absence of a large corpus of literature on a country's traditional medicine tends to depend on whether the country is colonized and the extent to which the colonizers have outlawed the practice and consequently the documentation of traditional medicine. In the nineteenth century and most of the twentieth, Europeans were championing colonization, exploitation, and commerce. Janzen (1974-1975), in a discussion of Belgian colonial policy in the Congo, notes that "indigenous therapeutic practices were never mentioned within colonial manuals or laws. These laws sought only to establish European-modelled institutions regardless of what may have pre- or co-existed in African society" (p. 109). Ralph Schram's *A History of Nigerian Health Services* (1971) never mentions the traditional healers who were serving the people prior to the colonizing exercises of the British (cited in Harrison, 1984).

During the early part of the twentieth century, there was a shift of emphasis from the conquest of Africans, Asians, Latin Americans, and Oceanic peoples to the control and co-optation of these peoples. This shift in emphasis was aimed at the maintenance of law, order, and economic growth. Thus, non-Western beliefs and values were ignored. The medical beliefs and practices of most non-European peoples were considered primitive, savage, and barbaric; they were considered not medicine, but magic, religion, or witchcraft (Seijas, 1975). As a result, laws were promulgated to criminalize the practice of traditional medicine.

A few decades later, Bronislaw Malinowski (1954) and A. R. Radcliffe-Brown (1952) learned that religious rites, beliefs, and practices served to maintain order in society and to regulate individual and group sentiment and behavior. Religious rites have a specific social function, namely, to regulate, maintain, and transmit from one generation to another the sentiments on which the constitution of the society depends. "Generally speaking, religious ceremonies take believers away from the mundane affairs of life, sometimes by presenting exhilarating experiences" (Harvey, 1988, p.103). Religion is critical to an understanding of the spiritual dimension of health, which in turn is pivotal to the maintenance of the psychosocial dimension of health. In other words, there is more to health care than medical care. Health care delivery systems do not exist in and of themselves, but as parts of larger sociocultural wholes. Health care systems comprise a set of resources that may serve nonmedical as well as medical goals.

A reassessment of the disease-focused approach to health care has led many social and behavioral scientists to adopt a social action approach to health care delivery, particularly in Southern countries. This means that the views of the community (the emic perspective) are now believed to be as important as, if not more important than, "scientific" views (etic perspectives). Medical and health beliefs and practices that had in the past been deemed superstitions are being reassessed and given fresh interpretations. These beliefs constitute symbolic representations of various realities, many of which are non-Western. Maladies resulting from hot-cold imbalance, the dislocation of internal organs, impure blood, unclean air, moral transgression, interpersonal struggle, and humans' relation to the spirit world are now seen as different manifestations of some general reality. When people define physical or emotional symptoms within a traditional taxonomy, they are likely to seek help in the traditional health care system. Thus, as Nigerian health education specialist Z. A. Ademuwagun (1974-1975) indicates, Nigerians in the Ibarapa district of Oyo state use traditional healers for excessive worry, sleeplessness, malaria, yellow fever, and snakebite. T. A. Lambo (1978), retired deputy director general of the World Health Organization (WHO), faults the Western medical practitioner as being "invariably preoccupied with immediate natural causes, almost to the exclusion of the causal relations between conflicts and irregularities in the field of social relations on the one hand and disease or misfortune on the other." Traditional healers generally became a focus of research because they were thought to have knowledge about herbal concoctions that may be useful in treating such health problems as hypertension, diabetes, and other chronic diseases that Westerners have found difficult, if not impossible to cure (Harrison, 1974).

Traditional Healing Concepts

The belief that a state of balance exists within the individual on the one hand and between the individual and the environment on the other is a concept that is true for all traditional healing modalities worldwide. How this concept is operationalized varies among cultures and hence among different traditional healing systems. African traditional medicine seeks to secure and maintain a balance among the individual, elements of nature, and the heavenly bodies. Within the individual, a balance is maintained among organic disorders, physiological disorders, and social conflicts. This balanced state is, in turn, balanced with elements of nature - earth, fire, water, air, and metal. Finally, balance is sought with the heavenly bodies - the sun, moon, and stars.

Organic and physiological disorders are concepts that are familiar to allopathic medicine. Social conflict is also a familiar allopathic concept in understanding psychological disorders. Expressions such as "He gets under my skin" and "She makes me sick" are examples of manifestations of social conflicts. In the African traditional healing context, an understanding of social conflict is pivotal to curing a person who has become ill. This is where the healer deals with the *ultimate* cause of an illness: who or what caused it, and why. The *proximate* cause, or specific etiology, tells only how it happened, not why it happened. For people who believe in this concept of disease nosology, knowledge of germ theory is useful only for explaining the medium through which health problems manifest themselves.

Ultimately, the origin of the disease or malady must be explained and dealt with. The body, mind, and environment must function in harmony for the individual to experience optimum health. In fact, in homeopathy, disease symptoms are considered good indications of the body's attempt to heal itself. For example, shivering in cold weather is the body's attempt to generate more heat in order to increase the core temperature of the body, and one should potentiate the shivering process rather than stop it; high fever is the body's attempt to make the environment uncomfortable for germs; and the cold and clammy skin of a person in shock is the result of the smaller blood vessels' diverting blood to the vital organs for the person's survival. The human body's ability to regulate itself naturally, as well as to synchronize the functions of its various organs and vessels to maintain a state of balance and harmony, is a basic principle of traditional medicine. It is this natural mechanism for dealing with states of balance and imbalance that traditional healers have always understood and attempted to maintain.

Traditional medicine is a desirable part of a nation's formal health care system, particularly in rural areas. Some 70% of the Western-trained doctors in Nigeria live in six cities (Benin, Enugu, Ibadan, Ife, Lagos, and Zaria) (Osuntokun, 1975), and most of the country's rural population relies solely on traditional practitioners to care for their health needs (Oyebola, 1986). Therefore, it behooves health professionals to examine the strengths and weaknesses of traditional medicine, so that they can promote its strengths and discourage its weaknesses for the benefit of the people who believe in it and use it.

Traditional medicine has paralleled the practice of Western allopathic medicine in a number of ways. In 1879, Robert Felkin, a British medical missionary traveling in Baganda (modern-day Uganda), reported a high level of medical and health practice. He saw the successful performance of cesarean sections, with antiseptic techniques, by a native surgical team. He also saw experiments devised to discover a cure for a local epidemic (J. N. P. Davis, 1959). Although Felkin witnessed this only two years after Joseph Lister advocated the use of antisepsis for surgery in London, it was clear to Felkin that the team's "surgical technique" and "public health experiments" were a part of the tradition of the Baganda. This suggests that the use of antisepsis by the traditional healers of Baganda predates its use by allopathic surgeons.

Other contributions made by traditional healers to health care delivery include the discovery of many herbal remedies, including *Rauwolfia serpentina*, a medicinal plant known as snakeroot, whose active ingredient, reserpine, is used today as a tranquilizer and hypotensive agent (Basch, 1990); *Erythropleum guineense*, identified from the bark of the sasswood tree, a powerful laxative substance (Foster, 1963); and *Periwinkle vinca rosea*, an herb containing insulin, which is used in the treatment of diabetes mellitus (Foster, 1963; Teller, 1968).

In addition to their contributions in the use of medicinal plants, traditional healers have been very successful in treating psychosomatic disorders. Lambo (1961) provides an example of healers' (*babalawos* of Nigeria) ingenuity:

> A toad is tied to the penis of the bed wetter. If the child urinates, the heat from the urine wakes up the toad, who then begins to croak. The croaking of the toad wakes up the child. The similarity of this device to the modern anorectic machine is evident. The modern anuretic machine delivers a shock to the bed wetter on urinating. Behaviorally speaking, the electric shock and the croaking of the toad function as negative reinforcers.

Another example was shared by a British-trained physician from Mauritius who attended a lecture I gave on traditional medicine in June 1991 as part of the Boston University School of Public Health summer certificate program titled Health Care in Developing Countries. He recounted the story of a Nigerian soccer player who had suffered a compound leg fracture in the 1970s and was healed by a traditional bonesetter. When the limb healed, however, it was shorter than the uninjured limb, such that the patient was left with a limp. The patient went back to the traditional healer to seek a solution and was instructed as follows: He was to ask a friend or relative to go to the river with him and tie him up in the part of the river with the heaviest wave for one hour every day. At the end of six months, the patient's broken leg was back to its normal length - the strength of the river's current had realigned the bone properly. This approach was, of course, very different from the one that would have been taken in an allopathic system, in which the bone would have been rebroken in a hospital and reset. Although it would be naive to suggest that traditional medicine is a panacea for the health problems of Africans, it certainly has the proven evidence to improve the health care delivery system significantly for many people.

An understanding of the function of traditional medicine in any culture must begin with an understanding of the culture and its history. This is a challenge for behavioral and social scientists who have an interest in solving the health problems of developing countries. As a result of the renewed interest in traditional medicine, partly because of the primary health care movement and, more recently, the child survival revolution, the integration concept is now in vogue. Even given the problems that have been identified in the integration of traditional medicine with allopathic approaches (Pillsbury,1982), international donor agencies concerned with primary health care, child survival, and safe motherhood have all displayed interest in such integration in their programs. However, often these agencies view the potential contributions of traditional medicine as very limited. On the strength of their economic resources, such agencies have dominated health policy and practices in the Third World since World War II (Justice, 1987). Along with their influence and funding resources have come policy guidelines and priorities that have always promoted allopathic hegemony.

Major difficulties with government policy arise from perceptions and definitions of traditional medicine. Murray Last (1986) observes:

> Though within most nations there are usually a large number of medical subcultures, each with its own characteristics and structure, policymakers often have in mind apparently a single, paradigmatic culture from which they generalize about "traditional

medicine." Inevitably such stereotypes are likely to reflect political conditions - as of course happened under colonial rule when traditional healers were categorized as "witches." (p. 4)

Issues of Integration

Failure to historicize traditional healing has resulted in misguided efforts by allopaths, albeit with sincere intentions, to address the formalization of traditional healing within the health care system. Historically, traditional healers were specialists at a time when allopaths were generalists. Healers specialized in diagnostics, maternal and childcare, bone setting, and so on. The earliest attempts by governments to legitimize and confirm traditional healers encountered difficulties when physicians, who were generalists, proposed to traditional healers, who were specialists, that they should all come together under one umbrella as traditional healers. The impetus for such unification was to standardize traditional practice rather than for political and social leverage, as in the case of allopaths. Because the bonesetters could never understand the wisdom of a forced marriage with maternal and child health specialists (even though a few might specialize in both), unification never materialized. In cases in which unification has occurred today, it is for the same reason as Western allopathic unification - political leverage within a society. It should be noted, however, that approaches to specialization have changed for both traditional healers and allopaths. Whereas physicians now train to become specialists, traditional healers train to become generalists. These transitions have been fueled by the desire to maximize economic leverage.

Physicians continue to be suspicious of traditional healers because, they assert, healers blame their patients when the patients fail to recover. In their defense of standardization, physicians claim to assume responsibility for the deaths of patients by coming together with their colleagues (in professional standards reviews) and discussing how to learn from mistakes so as not to repeat them. Physicians see this not as professional secrecy, but simply as professionalism. However, when asked whether physicians would be satisfied with traditional healers' "professionalism" if healers were to meet regularly to discuss the outcome of fatal cases, physicians respond with a resounding no.

Thus, as perceived by physicians, professional responsibility comprises differing values, expectations, and interpretations for physicians and traditional healers. Few, if any, physicians will go to the family of a deceased patient to take responsibility for the death, even though that is what they expect of traditional healers. Moreover, many physicians fail to see that suggesting to the family of a patient who has just undergone an operation that "it is now up to the patient" or that "the patient's will to live is very important at this time" is a form of holding the patient personally responsible for his or her recovery and thus blaming the patient if he or she dies.

Physicians who insist that allopathic medicine is purely scientific, objective, and measurable are strongly opposed to keeping score cards that might compare their professional skills with those of their peers, on the grounds that there are other factors that make medicine less objective and measurable, and perhaps less scientific. Yet physicians accuse healers of being unscientific and insist that healers be subject to individual, objective, and scientific evaluation - the very measures of professional performance to which they are strongly opposed for themselves.

It seems quite apparent that in medicine, there are certain levels of nonscientific, subjective, and perhaps even "magical" practices. The "scientific" aspects and the "human aspects" jointly potentiate the possibilities of healing. Illich aptly notes this invoking of magic in allopathic practices in the epigraph that opens this chapter. The belief in magic within the Western "scientific framework" is not exclusive to medicine. Perhaps the most revealing of Western superstitions is the fact that many modern, shiny, glass-and-steel skyscrapers, financed, built, owned, managed, and occupied by the cream of Western bourgeoisie, have no thirteenth floors. Of course, the thirteenth floors are simply numbered 14 to deceive the witches, ghosts, and other evil spirits (Chinweizu et al., 1983, p.22)!

In 1977, the Thirtieth World Health Assembly adopted a resolution (WHA 30.49) urging governments to give "adequate importance to the utilization of their traditional systems of medicine, with appropriate regulations" (Akerele, 1984, p. 77). This became the stimulus that galvanized the World Health Organization to launch the global promotion of traditional medicine. It has been estimated that 80% or more of the world's rural population relies mainly on traditional medicines for health care needs (Bannerman et al., 1983). Three major recommendations have been made concerning (a) evaluation of traditional healing practices, (b) incorporation of traditional medicine as part of national health care systems, and (c) provision of training for traditional healers. To accomplish this goal, attempts have been made in different countries to find common ground for traditional medicine and allopathic medicine. The struggle to locate this common ground has led many to advocate for the integration of these two kinds of care systems. Such integration has been promoted by many respected organizations, including WHO and UNICEF, and scholars such as Bannerman et al. (1983), Lambo (1978), Akerele (1984), Pillsbury (1982), Maclean and Bannerman (1982), and Newman and Bhatia (1973).

Unfortunately, the implementation of integration has been based on a "donor-deficit model" for the traditional healers. The guiding belief is that traditional healers can be trained to "modernize" their healing practices by having allopathic professionals teach them what they do not know (that is, healers are assessed from a deficit model). In the process, allopaths find out what traditional healers know, so that their knowledge can be improved when applied to allopathic practice (healers become donors). The assumption is usually made that the healer, who supposedly needs some training, can make little or no contribution to improving the knowledge and practice of the allopath.

In discussions about the integration of traditional and allopathic health services, the traditional healer has rarely been viewed as a health provider with adequate or superior knowledge in certain aspects of health care that will be of benefit to the allopathic provider (physician) in a training session. The sources of traditional healers' concoctions and pharmacopoeia, however, are eagerly, even exploitatively, sought (Harrison & Cosminsky, 1976). Though deficient in some areas, traditional healers could be donors in other areas. Instead of receiving proper and due recognition for the areas in which they are known to be efficient and effective, healers are encouraged to surrender their herbal lore for the advancement of science.

Such mistakes in professional judgment do not end with allopathic physicians. Some behavioral and social scientists who believe in aspirin yet cannot explain how it relieves pain have demanded that traditional healers explain their medications before these scientists consider the medications valid, even though they are used for the same reason as aspirin, a strong belief in their healing power. This kind of inconsistent and one-sided judgment has led to reluctance and suspicion on the part of traditional health care providers. Instead of integration or cooperation based on mutual trust, respect, and collaboration, in most cases, the outcomes are distrust and suspicion.

As one explores the concept of integration further, three problems become evident. First, as stated above, the healer is seen as one who needs to be trained but who has nothing to contribute to training the allopath. Second, a conflict exists between didactic learning, which is how allopaths are trained, and experiential learning, which is how traditional healers are trained. Third, there is a lack of systematic protection of ownership of orally transmitted information, which is a vital form of intellectual and creative property in traditional medicine.

Integration has been more successful around childbirth practices than in other areas of traditional medicine (Pillsbury, 1982). This success has often been attributed to traditional birth attendants' not posing any serious competition to physicians in terms of their professional status, power, and resources (Green, 1988). In other cases of integration, governments have attempted to incorporate traditional healers into modern sector projects or programs (Pillsbury, 1982). These attempts almost always involve some kind of training for the healers to upgrade their knowledge. Unfortunately, the healers often receive training in the most basic and mundane tasks, such as mixing oral rehydration solutions, even though the healers would like to learn how to give injections and read X-rays (Green, 1988).

A training session designed for integration should be one in which both allopathic providers (particularly physicians) and traditional healers are trainers and trainees, because both have information to contribute and to gain. Integration should mean the involvement of healers in the planning, implementation, and evaluation of health service delivery to foster cooperation and participation. This does not necessarily mean moving the traditional healer to a hospital setting, any more than it should mean moving the physician to the healer's practice setting. Integration, for example, may mean appropriate referral from a physician to a bonesetter for fractures, as well as referral from an herbalist to an internist for appendicitis.

The second problem with integration is that of the often-ignored differences between allopathic and traditional healers in methods of knowledge acquisition, as applied to proposed training programs. Paramount among these are differences in perceptions of reality. Formal, didactic teaching is not usefully applied to traditional healing practice, in which learning in the apprenticeship mode (experiential learning) is more appropriate and culturally customary (Jordan, 1989). This is particularly true of the several training programs developed to "upgrade" the knowledge and skills of traditional birth attendants - the ubiquitous, taken-for-granted midwives (Maclean & Bannerman, 1982, p.201815).

The third problem with integration is that physicians have arrogantly requested that traditional healers share their knowledge about their treatments and medicines without setting up any systematic process to guarantee ownership of the information that is revealed. In Western culture, the protection of information, inventions, and discoveries, and their revelation, is guaranteed under copyright and patent laws. In a U.N. debate over how Southern nations are to be rewarded for contributions to plant species, Henry Shands, a U.S. delegate, argued that without a strong patent law, there is no incentive for people to investigate the possible superior medicinal properties of plant species (Simons, 1989).

Although patent and copyright laws are not customary in oral tradition, revelation of information within this context has always been protected. One method of such protection has been for healers to reveal information only to one or two protégés. Thus, open, widespread revelation is an allopathic phenomenon and should carry with it the protection and rewards that go with it or, alternatively, a culturally appropriate modified version. When traditional healers possess the knowledge to discover, create, and use compounds of superior medicinal properties, such information should not be shared with others in the absence of some system guaranteeing that the original sources of such information or medication are protected and/or appropriately rewarded for their revelation. Although healers may not articulate such a right, it is a basic human desire to be assured of ethical protection of these fundamental principles regarding information sharing and proprietorship, regardless of the pattern of knowledge acquisition.

Such protection and rights of ownership are paramount in promoting open information sharing and true reciprocity between and among health providers and policy makers. The resistance of physicians to sharing information with traditional healers could be considered an example of such protection. It should, however, be noted that such reluctance about integration is not unique to physicians. It is also true of medical anthropologists, medical sociologists, health educators, and other public health professionals. However, the stakes are much higher for the public when healers, both allopathic and traditional, do not cooperate with each other to maximize health coverage for the people, so that the public might benefit from the best of both worlds.

International health professionals will have a better appreciation of international health problems if they understand that treatment modalities, like diseases and disease patterns, are intricately tied to beliefs and values within cultures. As long as Africans successfully seek treatment from both allopathic and traditional healers, it is prudent to strive for mutual collaboration based on respect and trust between the two types of health providers. Perhaps the word should be *cooperation* instead of *integration*. The latter tends to conjure up resistance among those who interpret this process as an encroachment on their territory. This has been my experience during workshops and lectures on traditional medicine. If the PEN-3 method is used, beliefs and perceptions can be grouped into positive, existential, and negative domains, so that a complete and balanced view of a given modality can be obtained.

Implications for National Health Policy

An important factor contributing to successful national health policy in Southern countries is clear definition of the healing modalities. Such a definition should involve people from both allopathic and traditional healing systems. As Last (1986) advocates, traditional healers ought to organize themselves and seek professional status, in order not only to survive but to get their share of government support. Integration, registration, and professionalization, however, may be possible only after a period of official government recognition. Such recognition may take various forms, at various levels, in various contexts (Harrison, 1984) by *recognition*, I mean an array of relationships among traditional healers, government officials, and medical personnel that may range from private meetings to licensure. Healers, traditional or modern, are human and therefore may interact and exchange information as family members, friends, and professionals.

Policy makers should decide on communities' strengths and unmet health needs and then involve social and behavioral scientists, as well as community members, in health program planning, implementation, and evaluation. The community thus helps to define acceptable healing practices based on indigenous reasoning, which may be inexplicable in the Western context. Cultural diversity among peoples of different nations and the impact of such diversity on program replicability cannot be overemphasized. Community involvement is one strategy for acknowledging the impact of culture on a national health system. This is often realized when the individuals, families, and communities for whom a program is intended, as well as service providers (traditional healers), have the opportunity to be a part of the team that defines the health problems to be targeted and formulates their solution through the design of a particular health program. Sensitivity to traditional customs and social norms, and thus the cultural appropriateness of a program, is ensured through the participation of community members.

Allopathic health providers can learn from traditional healers, just as traditional healers can learn from allopathic practitioners. Understanding the components of a system of healing is critical to the ability to influence the health behavior of those who subscribe to that system. Consequently, Public health professionals, including health educators, should learn to be humbler about their profession and programs and should strive to become more understanding of others (Torrey, 1972). Some allopathic physicians have already started to utilize what they have learned from traditional healers. Some now place an amulet around a child's neck to ensure that the child returns for a follow-up visit, so the physician can maintain continuity of care until the patient is cured. Reciprocally, some traditional healers now send their fracture patients to have their bones X-rayed in a hospital. In child survival programs, the traditional wearing of beads around a child's wrist is being used for growth monitoring. Thus, there is already some level of cooperation.

Conclusion

One of the key primary health care providers in most Southern countries is the traditional healer. Because traditional medicine is based on cultural and traditional values, it is important for health educators to affirm and legitimate this modality within the formal health care system. Ignoring traditional medicine is tantamount to ignoring the cultural impact of health and disease in these societies. After all, one cannot sincerely address health care delivery in Africa without giving adequate coverage to traditional medicine. Social and behavioral scientists who are interested in health care delivery in Southern nations should devote adequate time to an exploration of the past, present, and future contributions of traditional healers to health care delivery in these countries. This was done, for example, when the WHO Global Programme on AIDS and Traditional Medicine Programme convened an informal consultation in Geneva in February 1989 to review the status of research and services in traditional medicine as applied to HIV infection and AIDS (World Health Organization, 1989).

Social and behavioral health scientists must be willing to experiment with various forms, at different levels, and with definitive contexts in order to establish and promote proper communication with traditional and allopathic health providers. Communication and cooperation must prevail if there is to be an optimal working relationship between these forms of health services. Therefore, social and behavioral scientists have critical roles to play in improving global health care policies and systems, and it is vital that they work with traditional healers to ensure the provision of adequate health care systems in Southern nations. Such systems will ensure that Africans have available, accessible, acceptable, and affordable health services and will allow all Africans to benefit from the best of both worlds (Akerele, 1986).

NOW:

My Conversation with Stella Iwuagwu and Randy Shine

Cultural and Professional Identity - Positionality

Airhihenbuwa: See my intro in chapter one

Iwuagwu: I'm a daughter. My late father was a very loving man who imbued so much love in me. My mother is hardworking, and I inherited many of my herbalism skills from her. I'm a mother of two loving children, a sister, an aunt to many nieces and nephews, and a friend to many friends who kept me alive. I'm a mentee and a mentor, mentored by incredible people, including Professor Airhihenbuwa. Professionally, I'm a public health educator and social entrepreneur. I'm the Executive Director of the Center for the Right to Health, and a farmer at Sustainable Demonstration Farms, which I hold dearest among all my achievements because it reshaped my life. I'm Nigerian, American, and a global citizen. I'm a lifelong learner and researcher.

Shine: I like to say I define myself based on biological and social experiences. I'm a Black man/African American, and how I navigate society comes from that perspective. I live in Philadelphia, a city known for its grit and tenacity. My father was a prominent pastor, and I grew up in a religious household. As a Black man, I wrestle with intercultural issues and challenges that African Americans face within our community and issues we face from outside our community. My early career was in academia. Today, I'm a professional magician. I travel around the country performing on college campuses, resorts, corporate, and private events.

The Healing Power of Magic

Airhihenbuwa: I've always seen magic as a form of healing, especially when you perform for children in hospitals. It reminds me of traditional healing and how it helps people imagine and heal."

Shine: Magic is indeed healing. A study conducted by the University of Cape Town on the College of Magic (A non-profit Art organization that teaches magic to children) showed how learning magic boosted confidence and imagination for children in townships. Graduates from the program gained skills that transformed their lives. Magic helps people believe in the impossible. I've performed for patients in hospitals, and the feedback is always that it lifted their spirits. Another study showed magic helped reduce anxiety in patients. I've had audience members tell me my performance helped them through grief and trauma. One young man I once taught magic to as a child, who had congenital heart issues, recently attended my show and told me how my attention to him and teaching him years ago gave him a sense of normalcy. Magic provides emotional relief. In our Black communities, where mental health is still taboo, magic offers some relief and can serve as a bridge.

Airhihenbuwa: Branding matters. Just like France brands its coffee, even though the country has no coffee farm, we must embrace and brand our own healing practices. Even our clothing and art have been rebranded from external sources. Our imagination and our identity must guide us in reclaiming and owning these practices.

Shine: People say I'm more than a magician, I'm a storyteller. My magic effects metaphors for life and living. *I'm an African griot using magic to ignite imagination. 'Abracadabra' means 'I create as I speak.' Imagination leads to transformation.* I joke that I'm 'Black Jesus,' but it's intentional, to challenge dominant imagery and reclaim spiritual imagination. Magic connects people. A magic show on a cruise ship becomes a catalyst for strangers to bond. That's the healing power of community.

Airhihenbuwa: Arts like magic deserve the same platform as the visual arts in healing. Evidence doesn't only come from science, it also comes from belief, community, and experience.

Shine: Although magic is a form of entertainment, I also view it as an art form. In my formal shows, I present "tricks" in a way that expresses concepts and shares a bit of history. I always believe that artists can speak in ways that others cannot, because we have that freedom and latitude, even when the topic is controversial, with little to no consequence. I'm proud to help other Black performers explore the history of Black magicians, intertwined with American history. I'm 100% unapologetically Black in thought, expression, and movement. I lost both my parents in the past two years. I am fortunate to have elders, like you, Dr. Airhihenbuwa, who offer guidance and reflection. I've learned from you that I must become *comfortable with being uncomfortable.*

Food as Healing for Mind, Body, and Spirit

Airhihenbuwa: You used food as a path to healing after your accident. Your experience shows how returning to one's roots can inspire others.

Iwuagwu: My journey was shaped by both allopathic and traditional medicine. After a spinal cord injury, I was paraplegic and on 21 medications while in the US. I returned to Nigeria due to a family tragedy- the loss of my younger sister from complications of childbirth. I blamed the health system and health workers, even making a documentary, *Failed by Angels*, criticizing them. But over time, I saw the truth: the healthcare system is overwhelmed and under-resourced, and patients cannot get quality healthcare under those circumstances, especially with a very sick population. I examined the environmental and social conditions that are making people sick. I realized that food insecurity was a major culprit. People who had access to healthy food had better immune systems and could fight off infections. I remembered how we supported people with HIV through food-based immune support. I was also concerned by the high rate of chemical applications in food production and felt that this is also a major concern. I was not comfortable buying food from the market. So, I started an organic homestead garden. I was a proactive gardener; I crawled to weed and plant every morning. I eat from my garden. The healing was profound. I lost weight, and my pain lessened. I went from 21 medications to 3. This shifted my focus from healthcare systems to food and environmental health.

I revived traditional farming methods. Today's food is filled with chemicals. So, I started edible landscaping, encouraging people to plant what they eat and exercise through farming. It reconnects us with nature and improves health. Our grandparents' diets and farming habits were deeply nutritious. Herbs like scent leaf, lemongrass, bitter leaf, and ginger are powerful. Yet *we've been conditioned to reject our own healing traditions in favor of Western pills.* Now, we even import capsules made from our herbs. We must return to our roots.

Iwuagwu: For the future, we need African researchers to validate our herbal knowledge through rigorous clinical trials. I work with the Integrative Medicine Association in Nigeria, where we have professors of medicine, homeopathy, acupuncture, herbalists, and spiritualists; it is a wide tent. We respect and learn from each other. I learned about 'spiritual' plant called *Newboldia laevis,* it is used as a border or fence plant in most cultural homes and is believed to have spiritual application and other healing properties; unfortunately, people cut them down out of ignorance. It is difficult to find it now. We've lost so much traditional knowledge because of the shame imposed by colonial and religious mindsets. We need to research and document these traditions and honor them.

Africans love to dance. I use dance as therapy. I encourage individuals and families to dance. They can even start dance competitions, cook and eat together, which improves social connections, mental and physical health. I promote ancient grains like fonio (acha), finger millet (Tamba), low glycemic gluten-free grains that can serve as alternatives to imported wheat. *Food is healing and growing it can create financial empowerment.* I tell kids, 'Money grows on trees.' Plant pawpaw, coconuts, turn farming into entrepreneurship. Our health framework must include the financial dimension. I teach students to farm, eat well, and sell produce. That's healing, too.

Final Thoughts

The conversation centered on imagination, community, and the reclamation of African healing traditions, whether through magic, food, farming, or herbal medicine. Healing must be holistic: mental, physical, spiritual, and financial. The future lies in integrating traditional practices with evidence-based validation, while encouraging communities to believe in and build their own paths to wellness.

Chapter 5

African Women's Health and the Confluence of Patriarchal and Western Hegemonies

THEN:

> The true worth of a race must be measured by the character of its womanhood.
>
> Mary McLeod Bethune, "Century of Progress of Negro Women," 1933

Whereas in one culture an individual's opportunities to make decisions that ultimately shape his or her destiny may rest with the person's level of independence in both the family and society, in other cultures it is an individual's level of autonomy that determines such decision-making ability. Autonomy is often confused with independence, especially when the discussion focuses, cross-culturally, on the issue of social and economic freedom for women. Autonomy does not necessarily require that one be independent of one's family or partner, if one's role and contribution in society are duly recognized and valued economically, culturally, and socially. The issues of autonomy and independence undergird the differences in how Western women and African women view the plight of women in general.

One of the issues related to the role of men in women's oppression is the economic valuation of women's contribution to family stability and growth. When it is a question of serving their own interests, men conceive of work only in terms of payment, but when it is a question of valorizing the rights of women, they find it absurd that women demand to be paid for their services (needless to say, the housewife works even if she is helped by a maid, just as men in the workplace give to their subordinates all the burdensome tasks) and appeal to the duties of love. Thus, the ambiguity of giving and of duty is manipulated at will by men according to the circumstances (Minh-ha, 1991).

African women are no different from Western women in terms of working long hours and receiving few or no remunerative and/or social supports and rewards commensurate with their labor. Having to work under these conditions, women naturally have the need and desire to seek efficient and effective ways to use available human and material resources to reduce their workload and enjoy some leisure time during the day. The differences between African and Western women in general lie in the opportunities and liberty they have to use such resources (e.g., human resources such as children or material resources such as domestic technology) as well as to manage the environment (such as family expectations) to achieve life's goals. For example, many African women do not have at their disposal domestic appliances, such as machines for pounding *fufu* or *cassava,* or individual and/or accessible neighborhood washing machines and dryers, which could relieve them of some of the burden of their endless, arduous tasks. Yet men can always purchase motorized vehicles (as opposed, for example, to bicycles) for transportation and can even afford luxury items such as stereos, televisions, and VCRs. In fact, when Yam Poundo (a machine for pounding yam) became available at a reasonable price (less than the price of an average stereo) in Nigeria in the early 1980s, many men who could afford one would not buy one for their wives because they believed that the machine did not pound yam as smoothly as could a woman using mortar and pestle. Some of their wives agreed. This seeming complicity of the wives can be seen as the propagation of values internalized over time, even though such values may not serve one's interest. However, it should be noted that there will always be initial skepticism in adopting a new product, particularly when it challenges the perceived usefulness of traditional practice.

Those men who bought and encouraged their wives to use the machine did so after they found out that the pounded yam they ate in their favorite restaurants was made in such machines. Thus, even when the new technology was finally adopted, it was not adopted because of its benefits in time effectiveness and efficiency for wives, but because husbands realized that it would not compromise their interests (the taste of the yam). This is an attempt not to demonize maleness, but rather to problematize the way in which patriarchal domination is nurtured and reinforced even by men who may be committed to the struggle for gender equality.

Where the Western woman complains of being doubly oppressed, the Black woman of Africa suffers threefold oppression: patriarchal domination by virtue of her sex, capitalist exploitation by virtue of her class, and appropriation of her country by colonial or neocolonial powers by virtue of her race (Thiam, 1986). The historical terrain of oppression perpetuated by men on women has tended to parallel the patterns of cultures that otherwise embody totally different values and meanings. Such a seemingly synchronized timeline among and between different cultures in constructing and executing patriarchal hegemony is captured by Achebe (1987):

> The original oppression of women was based on crude denigration. They caused Man to fall. So, she became a scapegoat. No, not a scapegoat which might be blameless but a culprit richly deserving of whatever suffering Man chose thereafter to heap on her. That is the Woman in the Book of Genesis. Out here, our ancestors, without the benefit of hearing about the Old Testament, made the very same story, differing only in local colour. At first, the Sky was very close to the Earth. But every evening, Woman cut off a piece of the Sky to put in her soup pot or, as in another version, she repeatedly banged the top end of her pestle carelessly against the Sky whenever she pounded the millet or, as in yet another rendering - so prodigious is Man's inventiveness - she wiped her kitchen hands on the Sky's face. Whatever the detail of the Woman's provocation, the Sky finally moved away in anger, and God with it. Well, that kind of candid chauvinism

> might be OK for the rugged taste of the Old Testament. The New Testament required a more enlightened, more refined, more loving, even, strategy - ostensibly, that is. So the idea came to Man to turn his spouse into the very Mother of God, to pick her up from right under his foot where she'd been since Creation and carry her reverently to a nice, corner pedestal. Up there, her feet completely off the ground, she will be just as irrelevant to the practical decisions of running the world as she was in her bad old days. The only difference is that now Man will suffer no guilt feelings; he can sit back and congratulate himself on his generosity and gentlemanliness. Meanwhile, our ancestors out here, unaware of the New Testament, were working out independently a parallel subterfuge of their own. Nneka, they said. Mother is supreme. Let us keep her in reserve until the ultimate crisis arrives and the waist is broken and hung over the fire, and the palm bears its fruit at the tail of its leaf. Then, as the world crashes around Man's ears, Woman in her supremacy will descend and sweep the shards together. (p.89)

The gender inequity in African culture is a process that begins in the family and is perpetuated through cultural values and beliefs and institutionally reinforced throughout society. For example, the father who has three sons and three daughters but only enough resources to provide a solid foundation for the future well-being and social and economic independence (e.g., education) for four of his children may choose to do so for all three sons, no matter their birth order, and then choose one "lucky" daughter. Already, the boys are ahead, thus marking the beginning of their privileged position. Everything else that follows serves only to perpetuate the foundation that has been established in the family. In the traditional African philosophy, knowledge obtained through Western formal education is a power that should be reserved only for males, who will inherit the land, thus placing women at great disadvantage (Njoku, 1980). Even when equal foundations are established for all the family's children, regardless of sex, landownership issues remain a measure of inequality between men and women. The point here is not to demonize maleness and romanticize femaleness, but to illustrate the historical genealogy of the nature of patriarchal domination in many African cultures. This is the only way to address the dismantling of the tools of women's oppression. Such dismantling will require the collective effort of men and women. The involvement of men is critical in the promotion of equity through, among other things, the elimination of different forms of oppression of women. This is why women of African descent differ from White feminists in women's emancipatory projects. As bell hooks (1993) has stated, "I believe that men must be part of the feminist movement, and they must feel that they have a major role to play in the eradication of sexism. The term `women's movement' reproduces the notion that somehow feminism is this plantation that only women should labor on" (p.37).[1]

Women in general suffer oppression in a male-constructed world, but the women of Africa suffer additionally from being left out of the women's struggle by White women. Most analysts who have evaluated the oppression of women in Africa have tended to view women only in the role of wives. White feminists, for the most part, do not engage in a dialogue on the contradictions that constitute and shape the role of Black women in a family context, as sisters, aunts, or daughters (Amos & Parmar, 1984). African women's agency is invoked as "daughter" and "sister," yet these dimensions tend to be missing in attempts, particularly by Westerners, to gauge the praxis of women's rights in African countries. What is often highlighted is female circumcision or mutilation, a practice that is opposed by many Africans, particularly feminists/womanists, as they are better able to situate such oppositional projects within the cultural framework under which this practice is promoted. Amos and Parmar (1984) note: "Many white feminists have argued that as feminists they find it very difficult to accept arranged marriages which they see as reactionary. Our argument is that it is not up to them to accept or reject arranged marriages but up to us to challenge, accept, or reform, depending on our various perspectives, on our own terms and in our own culturally specific ways" (p.15). Dawit and Mekuria (1993) assert:

> A media campaign in the West will not stop genital mutilation. Westerners and those of us living in the West who wish to work

> on this issue must forge partnerships with the hundreds of African women on the continent who are working to eradicate the practice. Neither Alice Walker nor any of us here can speak for them; but if we have the power and the resources, we can create the room for them to speak, and to speak with us. (p. A27)[2]

Some observers have pointed out that African feminists have not imposed facial surgery (or is it facial mutilation?) on Western feminists as a cultural project. Cosmetic surgery for beauty enhancement is tied to Western normative standards of beauty. This standard is largely dictated by male preferences and expectations of beauty. For example, breast augmentation is clearly a glaring case of female internalization of the male gaze. Some might argue that both breast augmentation and facial mutilation are voluntary. However, there is nothing voluntary about individual actions that are taken to fulfill societal expectations, whether such expectations are metaphysically enforced by the individual or directly promoted and implemented by the community. To suggest that facial surgery/mutilation is voluntary, as opposed to circumcision/genital mutilation, is to believe naively that societal forces do not significantly shape human behavior. One can only imagine the number of people who would undergo facial, breast, or other bodily transformation/mutilation if such services were free or inexpensive. Excision and infibulation are deeply rooted in the societies in which they are practiced, which is why protesting these practices by young women is often met with strong resistance on the part of older women (Thiam, 1986).

Pedagogical projects designed to subvert violence against women must historicize such violence within the context of culture and then affirm the efforts of feminists/womanists in that culture to subvert the violence, so that they can serve as legitimate voices and representation for the oppressed. It is important to note that passive resistance is a recognized and legitimate strategy that has been used effectively by the oppressed to subvert oppression. In other words, the oppressed have always believed that when one thing stands, another thing must stand beside it. The oppressed are not always powerless in the grassroots enterprise, as the notion of development participation would suggest. As Rahnema (1992) notes:

> Theirs is a different power which is not always perceived as such, and cannot be actualized in the same manner, yet it is very real in many ways. It is constituted by the thousands of centres and informal networks of resistance which ordinary people put up, often quietly, against the prevailing power apparatuses. Amongst others, it manifests itself in the reality of "taxpayers cheating the state, young people evading conscription, farmers accepting subsidies or equipment from development projects and diverting them to their own ends, technicians or repairmen working without permits or licenses, government-paid teachers using the classroom to denounce government abuses of power."(p.123)

Although American and European feminists can represent a voice for oppressed women in other societies, if they try to do so without affirming the work of their comrades in those societies, their work becomes a form of White female hegemony as well as cultural chauvinism. Such cultural chauvinism is the basis of the economic reductionism of Third World Women as found in the literature on women in development. Mohanty (1991b) notes: "The best examples of universalization on the basis of economic reductionism can be found in the liberal `Women in Development' literature. Proponents of this school seek to examine the effect of development on third-world women, sometimes from self-designated feminist perspectives" (p.63). One avenue where African women are constantly spoken for by their Western counterparts is through the ubiquitous nongovernmental organizations (NGOs).

> Fertility issues and third-world women's incorporation into multinational factory employment are identified as two of the most significant aspects of "women's worlds" in third-world countries. While such descriptive information is useful and necessary, these presumably "objective" indicators by no means exhaust the meaning of women's day-to-day lives. The everyday, fluid, fundamentally historical, and dynamic nature of the lives of third-world women is here collapsed into a few frozen "indicators" of their well-being. (Mohanty, 1991a, p. 6)

A number of the Western-based NGOs that are involved in health and development projects in African countries regularly deliberate over the most effective and efficient methods of promoting economic independence among women. One recommendation has been to train more women in income-generating activities for the sustainability of such projects as the child survival programs. "Gardening" is an occupation often recommended as suitable for women, but the nature of the work suggests that what is being recommended is farming. *Gardening* seems to be a more acceptable term because it romanticizes the labor involved. It suggests that the work is pleasurable and not as rigorous as farming. On the other hand, one cannot help but wonder if middle-class professionals, particularly women, are weary of being accused of encouraging their "sisters" to engage in farming. Whatever the reasons for recommending gardening, if such activity were being recommended for men, it would be called farming. Breastfeeding is another example of a practice that can be learned and promoted from within the culture, yet many NGOs now believe they have the requisite knowledge to train African women in how to breastfeed. There is little interest in challenging, for example, the promotion of infant formulas in these countries by Western-based corporations - a practice that has led to the abandonment of breastfeeding by some women for what is unfortunately believed to be a superior form of infant feeding. The NGOs that engage in teaching breastfeeding have assumed that if women from Southern nations do not breastfeed their babies, it is because they do not know how.

There are physiological events that occur only in womanhood (i.e., menstruation and menopause) that have been used by different cultures to fault women for the gender gap that has been established and perpetuated by men. Most cultures now embrace the medicalization of menstruation and menopause, such that the onsets of these natural events are marked by negativity. Both physical and emotional isolation and ostracism are commonly associated with the experiences of menstruating or menopausal women. Both experiences may be viewed as part of natural aging processes, but societal (Western medical) responses tend to suggest that many still believe they are pathological. Very little emphasis is placed on preparing young girls for menarche, and because of the negativity associated with and the medicalization of menopause, there is little interest in understanding how women in traditional cultures experience this life stage. W. Kamau (personal communication, 1993) interviewed some elderly Kenyan women and found that traditional women never experienced any of the typically expected psychomedical manifestations, such as hot flashes, irritability, and depression. Whether or not this is representative of the experiences of most women in Kenya and other African countries, it is clear that we are overlooking strategies employed by older women in Southern nations to live comfortably with the beginning phases of menopause. Rather than exploring the degree to which holistic traditional foods may buffer the so-called menopause syndrome, we place undue emphasis on medical interventions, such as estrogen replacement therapy. Instead of learning from traditional cultures about how women can positively experience these events, we have forsaken the cultural richness of human experiences in many Southern nations and are looking to the West for answers.

So profound are these dependency values that women themselves, having absorbed them, contribute to their promotion. In a culture constructed upon the complicity between the confluence of silence and submission, on the one hand, and philosophical misogyny, on the other, Chinese and other non-Western women not only are oppressed but also support their own oppression through the feelings of spiritual resignation that are dispersed throughout their societies (Chow, 1991). Western culture also contributes to the affirmation of womanhood only through the man's world. For example, a wife's adoption of her husband's name upon marriage is an alien custom that has been perpetuated by Western cultures in most traditional African societies (Mazrui, 1986). Traditionally, the women of Africa, my mother among them, retain their own names upon marriage. This is a legacy of the traditional African custom that helps to establish the individual within his or her own family lineage.

One aspect of the dimensions of health-seeking behavior that we have yet to explore concerns how the age gap between couples in Africa affects decision-making in the household. In cultures that place emphasis on seniority and aging in decision-making, a wife who is much younger than her husband does not necessarily have much decision-making power in the household. Such a hierarchy of authority is usually a function of cultural values and reality, albeit to the disadvantage of women. The promotion of equity and independence in this context may not prove as practical as an exploration of strategies to bridge the spousal age gap while educating the family and community about women's need for autonomy. People, mostly men, have often reduced the problem of women to a problem of complementarity, with the excuse that the liberation of Black people in general is far more important than the liberation of women (Thiam, 1986). For example, the debate about abortion is nothing more than religious persecution of women. The same churches that are ready to demonize women for making choices are curiously quiet and have passively reified both de facto and de jure polygyny - a choice that privileges men. Here are two practices that go against the teachings of the church, both of which can potentially threaten the life of a woman, but only one places the woman as the ultimate decision maker, and many people, including some women, want to stop her. According to Minh-ha (1991), "Freedom written by a man is understood immediately as freedom; the same word coming from a woman must be clarified if she doesn't want freedom to be understood as licentiousness" (p.122).

These are issues that must be considered on the macro level while we continue to deal with issues of individual and family health attitudes and behavior relative to health promotion and disease prevention. Throughout the nineteenth century, the British military in India was concerned only with maintaining an efficient and "healthy" army made up of men who had "natural" sexual desires that needed to be fulfilled (Amos & Parmar, 1984). In 1993, a similar policy was maintained by the U.S. military, as illustrated by the institutionalization of a regular supply of "healthy" Thai and Hawaiian female commercial sex workers for its men in uniform. Such commodification of women by governments is further evidence of postcolonial oppression.

Sexuality and the Discourse on Womanhood

The masculinized construction of blame and sexual being has placed the responsibility of controlling the spread of sexually transmitted diseases (STDs) on women. Strategies designed to control STDs such as AIDS must take cognizance of the social contexts in which they are operating and must fully appreciate the weight of cultural tradition in structuring the social/sexual relationships between men and women. The role of the supposedly 'supreme mother' earlier related by Achebe is particularly applicable here. They capture the extent to which traditional cultures tend to function on similar terrain with other cultures at any given time, even though the cultures may be operating at different locations. For example, women have been (and still are, in some cultures) held responsible for the sexes of their babies. Therefore, women's humanity is affirmed not only by their ability to have children but by their ability to have male children.

A discussion of the issue of sexuality in the African context is incomplete without mention of the role of men in providing a collective solution. For an indigent African American woman, sex may serve as barter for the financial support of a male partner (Mays & Cochran, 1988). A woman may place more value on securing food and shelter for herself and her children than on practicing safer sex. Moreover, negotiating condom use with a sexual partner, for example, sometimes creates the perception of promiscuity. If a woman asks her male partner to use a condom, she is implying either that he has been "immoral" or that she is amoral. If she implies that she has been sexually permissive, she may risk rejection by her male partner; if she implies that he has been sexually permissive, she risks his anger and outrage (Nichols, 1990). "In Nigeria, in each of the three major regional languages, Hausa, Igbo, and Yoruba, corresponding to different ethnicities, the phrase used for STDs may be translated as `women's diseases'" (Kisekka & Otesanya, 1990, quoted in Seidel, 1993, p.180). HIV prevention efforts need to recognize that sexual activity occurs within a social context, and that only interventions that are presented within an interpersonal decision-making framework may prove effective (Cochran, 1990; Mays & Cochran, 1988).

The reasons many women do not use condoms or do not negotiate condom use are related to sex role socialization and social class issues. In the United States, although it might seem that the inability of women to use or negotiate the use of condoms contributes to the maintenance of the imbalance in the male-female relationship, this female powerlessness is better understood in the larger context of the economic security, the sex-ratio imbalance, and the meaning of sex experienced by African American women (Cochran, 1990; Fullilove, Fullilove, Haynes, & Gross, 1990; Nichols, 1990). As Seidel (1993) notes, "Life-saving strategies, negotiation and self-expression need to come through demystification and empowerment, and through economic and political leverage" (p.181). This can be accomplished through government support for programs designed to address the disadvantaged position of women. If the PEN-3 model is used, positive, existential, and negative beliefs can be identified to ensure appropriate programmatic intervention. Examples of positive beliefs and actions in this context are cultural rituals in which women engage to prepare young girls for and to celebrate the passage into womanhood. An example of an existential practice is women's gender-related role as entrepreneurs, as evident in their success in commerce and trading, which, if equitably rewarded socially, culturally, and economically, can prove to be positive. An example of negative beliefs and practices is the custom of discouraging young girls from becoming high achievers because of concern over their difficulty in finding husbands.

Policy Implications

It appears that government policies target women only indirectly, through their children or their potential motherhood. A good example is the secondary focus on women found in child survival initiatives. Women are targeted in these programs to take responsibility for the improved health conditions of their children, not because women are considered worthy of such focus, but because their survival is inextricably tied to the survival of their children. Specific programs aimed at child survival, such as growth monitoring, oral rehydration therapy, breastfeeding/birth spacing, and immunization, rely on the involvement of women. Although the focus on child survival is laudable, a focus on family survival, particularly women's survival, is more crucial, because children are part of families, and the reality is that women are often the caretakers of their families.

Even when programs are designed to focus on the health concerns of women, they are still tied to the survival of children. An example is the Safe Motherhood Initiative, which, although admirable, particularly in light of the high rate of maternal mortality amongst Africans and African Americans, often does not address the social and environmental conditions that shape women's status in a community and society. Factors such as women's degree of autonomy within the family structure, leverage for resource acquisition such as property rights, and decision-making role relative to sex role and reproductive rights all mediate women's health status long before, during, and long after pregnancy. Therefore, improving the health conditions of women within the context of patriarchal hegemony should be the focus of health policies, so that women's health can be addressed as women's health rather than only as mothers' health. The issue is not that there is too much emphasis on the health concerns of children, but that there is too little emphasis on the health concerns of women.

Conclusion

The condition of women in a society can always be predicted by the overall status of women in that society. Therefore, programs aimed at improving women's health should commence with issues of equity for young girls. Low health status among women in a society not only affects the health of that society's children and youth but also serves as an obstacle to the full participation of women in the development process. The absence of policies directed toward ameliorating the inequity in women's health will eventually lead to failed programs for children and youth. In Chapter 6, I address the health concerns of children and youth.

Notes

1. Reprinted by permission of *Ms.* magazine, copyright 1993.

2. Copyright 1993 by The New York Times Company. Reprinted by permission.

NOW:

My Conversation with Nkiru U. Nzegwu and Titilayo A. Okoror

Cultural identity and professional identity

Airhihenbuwa: See my intro in chapter 1

Nzegwu: On the point of cultural identity, I am Ajie, from Isiokwe, Onitsha. Ajie is the title of all Isiokwe daughters. Interestingly, it is also the title of one of the seven highest-ranking chiefs of the Obi of Onitsha. This background is important because it lays the foundation of who I am, the rights available to me, and the historical knowledge I possess. The title connects me to a long, unbroken line of lineage daughters and the roles they've played throughout history. Lastly, I am also a mother and a grandmother. Professionally, being a SUNY Distinguished Professor is an accolade that marks the pinnacle of my career. I'm a philosopher by discipline, and I use philosophy to engage with African culture, making me also a cultural analyst. I'm an artist, I paint, and I look forward to returning more fully to that identity. I am not defined in a single way or by a single discipline, but rather by what I do.

Okoror: I am first a daughter, and that identity overshadows everything else in my life. I'm a first daughter, which comes with many responsibilities. I am also an aunt, a niece, and more recently, I have become the matriarch of my family as I've assumed the role of my mother. Professionally, I see myself as a teacher and scholar who is not confined to a specific discipline. I work across multiple spaces and domains in academia because I do not lock myself into any single field.

Cultural journey as an African woman

Airhihenbuwa: What has been your experience as a woman and an African Woman in the Academy?

Okoror: This is one of the most challenging questions. While reading the chapter and reflecting on my own identity, I thought about what it meant to be born into a culture with expectations for a first daughter. I have struggled with the concept of patriarchy, the very structure we pay homage to. As a girl child growing up in Nigeria, especially as a first daughter, I was expected to be industrious yet dependent on a man. I struggled with the tension between making my own decisions and deferring to a man's authority. This led me to feel the need to overexplain my choices. Today, I'm learning to stop overexplaining. I owe no one an explanation for my decisions. The more I reflect on my cultural identity, the more I realize how deeply it has shaped my professional life. When I was born, I came into the world with dreadlocks. In our tradition, specific rituals are performed to welcome such a child. My grandfather was a traditionalist, and I was raised in traditional African religion, not in the church. At age two, rituals were performed to acknowledge and celebrate my unique spiritual essence. I wore only white clothing to signify this. My father preserved the hair from my first haircut until his death. My cultural worldview and identity are full of contradictions. I am a woman whose birth signified independence and spiritual leadership, yet patriarchy demands that I defer to a man.

Nzegwu: My research work challenges the notion of patriarchy in African societies because of the epistemological framework that I use, and because that is not what I experienced. However, I've witnessed the growth of patriarchy and the erosion of cultural value, with the spread of evangelical Christianity. As its patriarchal doctrine and tenets are embraced, they are indigenized and represented as Igbo culture. Whilst traditionally Igbo women have been independent, increasingly they are expected to be submissive to their husbands on the misguided belief that this is how it was in the past. But the idea of Igbo women's submissiveness is a false one. Igbo women have always earned their own income, which was neither controlled nor shared with their husbands. Financial independence enabled them to make their own decisions based on their economic initiatives and trading realities, which their husbands always supported. This favorable social condition was fostered by three community-wide, powerful autonomous organizations that provided important platforms for different groups of women to protect their interests, assert their powers, and rebuff male dominance.

For most of the twentieth century up till the late 1960s, the power of mothers was reflected in the all-male Agbalanze society of Onitsha by the popularity of the title, Akunne, 'wealth of the mother.' An incident in the late 1970s further underscores the regulatory power of women. After a high-ranking chief publicly dishonored the officers of Ikporo Onitsha and died shortly afterwards, Onitsha women withheld burial rites until his family atoned for the disrespect.

Motherhood and Marriage in Nigeria before Colonization

Airhihenbuwa: Can you share some lessons to learn about the place of marriage and motherhood in your cultural spaces?

Nzegwu: My research demonstrates the centrality of motherhood and the ideology surrounding it. The deeply rooted nature of this ideology in African societies obstructed the formation of patriarchy and patriarchal structures. This is evident in the histories of many societies, Akan, Igbo, Yoruba, Hausa, Sotho, and others. Take Queen Amina of Zaria, for example, she was neither the first female ruler in Hausaland nor in Zaria. Her mother ruled Zaria before her, yet her mother's name is seldom mentioned. It is as if there is a conspiracy to erase mothers from history. Prior to European colonization, many communities in Africa were matriarchal, not patriarchal. Over 70% of African societies were matrilineal but are transitioning to patrilineal due to the impact of colonial era laws, and to Christianity and Islam. There is a profound shift in African cultural values that merits serious discussion.

Marriage and motherhood in Africa are conceptualized differently than in the West. In Africa, it is a means of expanding families, which is why both women and men can marry wives. One of my maternal aunts married a wife because she could not have children. This was entirely acceptable within the cultural logic of the society. Yet, when African and Western marriages are compared, the African side is swiftly downgraded while the Western is elevated. This is due, in part, to the contemporary dominance of Christian and Islamic ideologies that are devaluing African spirituality.

Okoror: In my research on Yoruba culture in Oyo State, I was drawn to the story of Efunsetan Aniwura, an Iyalode. She was a warrior and a leader. Her actions contradicted the gender norms I grew up with, in which women were to be submissive. She led warriors, and violated gender roles and expectations I thought were universal. Her story didn't fit the dominant ideology of being submissive, yet it was real and powerful.

African Culture and Motherhood

Nzegwu: As a cultural analyst, I had the opportunity to study societies. When people today refer to African traditions as patriarchal, they do not understand that this was not the case for most of the twentieth century. Men do not dominate women because they do not control maternal power and motherhood. Maternal power is a disruptive force. No man can assert authority over the being who gave him life. Mother's power is a mix of authority, compassion, and the capacity to bring people together. The ideology of motherhood does not rest on dominance. While mothers' law can be fearsome, it is resolute, not implacable. *African notions of motherhood are fundamentally different from the subjugated state of mothers that patriarchy propagates*. Patriarchal terminologies and frameworks introduced during colonial rule or through Christian and Islamic norms converge with feminist interventions to diminish the power of mothers. NGOs, in particular, have been complicit in perpetuating this narrative of African mothers as uninformed and misguided to align with donor expectations. The subordinate lens imposed on them frames African women as victims in need of saving. It successfully overlooks indigenous spiritual systems and the cultural autonomy that upheld women's rights and leadership for centuries.

Colonization and the Advent of Patriarchy in Nigerian Society

Nzegwu: We must debunk many assumptions about patriarchy that were propagated by colonial anthropologists because they clouded African women's conceptualization of themselves during the pivotal time of European colonization of Africa. The Aba Women's War of 1929 revealed much deeper issues about the male-privileging character of colonialism that the narrative on taxation does not. Taxation was a legitimate grievance because women were the money earners at the time and so had to foot the tax bill for their husbands and sons. But a more fundamental issue was the new warrant chief system, which appointed only men, and who exercised power in ways that were previously unknown, and that were disadvantageous to women. This societal power shift initiated by the colonial order upended the traditional gender balance in the society.

Igbo male historians focused only on the economic aspects of this uprising, overlooking the crucial shift in authority from women to men. Prior to colonialism, Igbo women could marry men or women and retain authority over their households. The person initiating the marriage, regardless of gender, was called 'Di,' a non-gendered term that defined the axis and line of inheritance. Colonial district officers and colonial laws disrupted the indigenous gender balance. They transferred women's personal properties to the male paramours they were living with. This was the beginning of a restrictive marriage system that prioritized male centrality, which became another nail in the coffin of Igbo women's autonomy. The colonial system also embedded new legal frameworks, including using the term 'manslaughter' rather than a gender-neutral or female-inclusive term, further marginalizing women within legal and cultural spaces.

Religion, Sexuality, and Patriarchy

Airhihenbuwa: We need to confront what Christianity and Islam have done in terms of reinforcing patriarchal norms. Men often embrace these religions because they serve as instruments for controlling women.

Okoror: I don't have a problem with submission; I have a problem with domination, they are very different concepts. As a Christian, I've found it challenging to reconcile some religious teachings with my deeper readings and understanding of the Bible. We need to engage women directly in conversations about Christianity and Islam, especially the contemporary ideologies they carry.

Nzegwu: One of our major challenges in Africa is ignorance of our cultures and spiritual values. Many Africans don't understand their own history, nor do they question the one that is pushed on them by colonialism and Christianity. Many do not know that women's problem with Christianity began with the Council of Trent in 895 AD, which banned women from being bishops or priests. That decision erased the powerful roles women played during Jesus's time and handed Christianity over to male authority. If the voices of women around Jesus had been preserved through history, Christianity today would look very different. We must remember what follows this monumental gender shift. Every book in the Bible was written by men, for men, and served a political purpose of subjugating half of humanity. We must interrogate both Christianity and Islam to expose their parochial nature. The problem is that we've universalized them, forcing African value systems to conform to what was always narrow and alien to us. If we want an African Christianity, we should look at Ethiopian Christianity and Coptic Christianity. It differs significantly from the white nationalist Christianity of European colonialism that emphasizes blue-eyed, blonde-haired Jesus.

African spirituality teaches us that the divine cannot be contained within four walls. It teaches us that fundamentally we are one, children of the first mother, Oma. The African mode of greeting, of "ibioma" (hugging), affirms our connection to the first mother, a recognition of the ties that bind us. Africa has advanced ethical and spiritual values, which Christianity and Islam undermine. The problem with these religions is that they stunt our potential and the blossoming of who we could become, as Africans, and as a global community.

The Future and Retelling African Women's Story

Airhihenbuwa: In my book *Healing Our Differences*, there's a chapter on women where I referenced a paper you, Nzegwu, wrote. You retold a story from Ifi Amadiume about a Western woman who went to Zimbabwe to teach community organizing, oblivious to the rich political history of women's organizing there.

It reminded me of figures like Margaret Ekpo, and the Igbo and Ibibio women who fought taxation, because women were the merchants, generating income, and taxation was a tool to control them. This chapter is really about retelling the story of African women and illuminating what agency truly means.

Okoror: Looking ahead, *we need to speak openly about the original cultures of Africa to educate others*. We don't need to call it feminism, because that's where a disconnect lies. For example, I'm often challenged for not using my husband's surname. I now respond by saying: 'I'm an Africanist. You're a colonial subject.' Before colonialism, women didn't bear their husbands' names. To move forward, we must know where we come from. Much of the younger generation doesn't want to be labeled 'difficult' or 'feminist.' They want to marry and have children, but on their own terms. Yet even that desire becomes difficult under current interpretations of 'wedlock.'

Nzegwu: We should leverage traditional practices to help women acknowledge and exercise their agency comfortably. Too many people have moved forward aimlessly because they were disconnected from their past, made to feel ashamed of it. When people call me a feminist, I take it as an insult. I believe there's nothing feminism can teach me. Feminism emerged within patriarchy and cannot see outside that paradigm. As Audre Lorde said, 'You cannot dismantle the master's house with the master's tools.'

Feminist ideas of equality, autonomy, and identity are embedded in patriarchal structures. We must critique feminism by learning from Africa. But that means Africans must know their own histories and cultures deeply. There's a new generation recognizing the limits of both patriarchy and feminism. They're looking to African value systems for guidance. Before feminism, there were African mothers. Our indigenous logic far surpasses the Western framework imposed during colonization. African men cling to patriarchal power because of their own sense of inadequacy, and they assert dominance when they feel most insecure. Women may accommodate or pretend to allow it, giving men the illusion of control, until the moment they shift.

Final Thoughts

The conversation focused on the tensions and contradictions between African women's cultural and professional identities, particularly regarding gender roles and societal expectations. The discussion underscored the importance of understanding and navigating these intersecting identities in our personal and professional lives. The real story in this reflection is not about patriarchy but about reclaiming African women's agency and spirituality before the incursions of Christianity and Islam. African spirituality was flexible and inclusive, with culturally enabled space for women to have broader choices and leadership. An example of such leadership is rooted in their status as mothers and birth position, especially for first daughters.

Chapter 6

The Cultural Production of Healthy Children and Youth

THEN:

Omonkaro - A child comes first.

Omonsigho - A child is more valuable than money.

Omonsefe - A child is more valuable than wealth.

Omonrotionmwan - A child is one's kin.

Omonragbon - A child is the world.

common names in Edo (Benin, Nigeria)

The naming of a child among the Edos of Nigeria, as well as many other groups in Africa, marks important cultural rituals within the family. Whether or not the naming of a child is marked by a ceremony, the selection of the name itself within the cultural context is never random. The name is designed to establish a specific historical trajectory as mediated by culture in the life of the family. The naming of children is symbolic of how different families try to reproduce themselves within their cultural codes and meanings. In this chapter, I define *youth* broadly as that period in an individual's life between childhood and adulthood. This period may encompass the preteen, teenage, and some post-teen years. In many African cultures, individuals at these ages are often referred to as young adults, because there is no term equivalent to *adolescent* or *youth* in many languages. A teenage person is usually referred to as *the young male child* or *the young female child*, which development professionals would refer to as the girl child or the boy child.

Children and youth foreground the constitution and meaning of the family (extended) in Africa. Therefore, an understanding of the role of children within African culture would be incomplete without an adequate contextualization of the construction and functions of the family as a cultural production. Many reasons have been offered in the literature to explain why Africans have many children, principal among which are that children provide a cheap labor pool in agrarian societies and that high infant mortality rates lead to the naturalizing of multiparous desire. Explanatory models that problematize high birth rates and attempt to offer solutions often focus only on economic outcomes. Although it is important to consider individual income levels when addressing family size and structure, it is equally important to balance economics with psychosocial, cultural, and spiritual dimensions of family formation. Although high infant mortality rates are undeniable in many parts of Africa, the desire to have many children is equally evident among non-agrarians who live in a "First World" environment within "Third World" societies. Thus, it is customarily understood that children form the core of what constitutes a family in most African contexts.

The Context of Family

In Nigeria, for example, most "professionals" (e.g., university professors) have larger families compared to their counterparts in Northern nations. It appears that not even "enlightened" professionals are immune to the cultural and psychosocial dictates of family size considered normative in their society. Surveys that constantly show the desire for fewer children among youths in secondary schools are quick to credit family planning programs for such reported projected expectations. Those who conduct the surveys, however, fail to recognize that similar expectations were expressed by many of today's parents who now have relatively large families. Expectations may be individually constructed based on social formations as understood at a particular point in time, but reality is collectively produced through many factors that are not always within the individual's immediate control yet influence them, both consciously and subconsciously.

The survival and thriving of the child is very much dependent on the survival and thriving of the family, particularly of the mother. It is said in Africa that an orphan is any child without a mother. To the extent that African mothers are the primary caretakers of children, mothers' well-being is inextricably bound to the well-being of children. Attempts to address children's well-being have led to such international health projects as child survival programs instituted under the strong support of international donor agencies. Some international health experts question the rationale for such vertical programs (vertical in the sense that they tend to stand alone), because these programs tend to overlook the myriad familial and contextual factors affecting the health of children. Furthermore, the factors that influence the desired number of children, how the wife/mother in the family negotiates her decisions, and the role that family support has on the financial responsibilities assumed by the husband/father all affect the number of children planned and whether those children will survive and have economic, cultural, and social support.

Health Issues and Services

Scarcity and unequal distribution of health facilities, along with limited economic and human resources, contribute to stark differences in infant and childhood disease rates across the globe. Of every 100 children born in Africa, 12 die within their first year. In contrast, the infant mortality rate is 1-2 out of 100 in the United States (except for the African Americans and other minorities) and other Northern nations (U.N. Development Programme, 1993). International health communities' efforts have been galvanized by increased understanding of the various benefits of child survival projects and the possibilities of removing various impediments that may thwart the potential achievements of these efforts. Two major child survival projects are the Expanded Program on Immunization (EPI) and programs promoting oral rehydration therapy (ORT). EPI was an ambitious effort to establish universal immunization against six common childhood diseases - measles, tetanus, pertussis, polio, diphtheria, and tuberculosis. ORT programs use a three-tiered strategy to treat life-threatening diarrhea in infants: (a) administering a simple sugar-and-salt solution, (b) continuing feeding during the episode, and (c) referring for care when appropriate. This low-cost approach replenishes fluids and electrolytes while also promoting preventive practices such as handwashing, breastfeeding, and immunization. Thus, ORT and EPI were complementary strategies.

However, regardless of the goodness of such projects' intent, the approach to the implementation of ORT programs and EPI epitomizes Western bias: Program administrators typically see only a problem to be solved and never acknowledge that the people involved may actually have their own method for overcoming it, given the right circumstances. Quite often, it is the circumstances that favor the disease's occurrence, progression, and recurrence that need to be checked. For example, David Werner (1989) warned against undue reliance on ORT packets, because this only creates dependence. Instead of placing emphasis on teaching parents how to mix oral rehydration solution at home, using local implements and ingredients, most ORT programs encourage the use of prepared solution packets. New Western-based industries were establishing rehydration solution manufacturing plants in African countries. One of the immediate negative consequences of these developments was the perception among many people that the ORT packets contain a cure for diarrhea rather than the premixed ingredients of a simple rehydration solution that can also be produced at home. This perception, in turn, caused many to lose confidence in the value of ORT. Given these challenges, culturally grounded approaches are essential. To address these concerns, the PEN-3 model was used as a guiding framework (the application of the model to child survival programs is discussed in Chapter 3).

Even when programs are successful in increasing the number of children who live beyond the age of 5, the years that follow are critical for these children's development, and this issue is often not addressed programmatically. In many societies, as youth enter adolescence, they are seen mainly in terms of their problems rather than as active members of society. In Southern countries, "street kids" are a current focus, as homeless children are in the West. Whereas proposed solutions in the West focus on engaging youth in activities that will keep them focused and free of boredom, in Africa, the emphasis should be on creating jobs (Fanon, 1968).

Cultural Construction of Youth

Adolescent is a term that is anchored in the medicalization of human growth and transformation. This term is a signifier that foregrounds such negative characteristics as out-of-control behavior, irresponsibility, indecisiveness, and fatalism. It is not surprising that many programmatic efforts directed at adolescents are designed to address a "natural deficit" that is believed to be inevitably present in this group. Thus, the word *adolescent* has several meanings - medical, cultural, political, legal, social, and historical. Whether adolescents are perceived negatively or positively, health promotion and disease prevention approaches directed toward them must be grounded in cultural realities.

In some societies, for example, a close relationship between a father and his son is believed to be optimal for the psychosocial well-being of the adolescent/youth. Such a relationship is commonly typified in the West by statements such as "My son is my best friend," and vice versa. Although close relationships between parents and children are also a goal in many African countries, such relationships translate to healthy and mutually enriching interactions, yet do not typify the notion of "friendship" as understood in the West. When I was growing up in Nigeria, the idea of (for instance) throwing a ball around with my father would have been as strange to me as it would have been to him. Yet I had the closest of relationships with my father, at the same time I had good friends among my peers. The need to engage in leisure activities with one's child, such as playing ball, is a Western concept that has no social value within the cultural milieu in which I was nurtured. Within the African context, parents are expected to remain parents; children are expected to have their friends within their peer group. This culturally based family interaction pattern is particularly salient given the average number of children in African families and the centrality of children in these families. As we recognize the economic benefit of having fewer children, we should also recognize the sociopsychological and cultural benefits of having many children within this context. Such contextualization of family size is vital if we are to debate and make recommendations about "appropriate" family size.

It should be noted here that there are certain disadvantages to having few children, even in the West. Increasing numbers of individuals in cultures in which small family size is the norm are tending to engage in professionalization of the extended family in the form of group therapy or support groups. Having no elders in one's family to advise one can also lead to professionalization of friendship in the form of counselors and/or therapists. The economic disadvantage (economic status being the core of Western notions of living) notwithstanding, there are notable social, psychological, and cultural benefits of having many children that we must not overlook in addressing the issue of family size in African cultural groups. The goal in deciding appropriate family size is to maintain a balance in all the important forces that shape the culture at a particular time.

The years that mark the bridge between childhood and adulthood are a very important evolutionary experience in individual growth and development. With so much negativity about the term *adolescent*, given its medicalized origin, perhaps a better term is *youth*. The youth of Africa today face more social and developmental challenges than their parents did. The often-conflicting value systems of their culture and of Western culture have complicated their decision-making and their ability to withstand environmental pressures to make healthy decisions. The confluence of the African top-down hierarchy of information flow and the top-down information flow within the school systems, which are borrowed from the West, has conditioned the youth to only receive information, never to produce it.

Youth may not be independent of family and societal institutions, such as schools, but they do function under the changing traditional values and customary practices of their environment.

When tradition is wrongly viewed as a static state, with the necessary knowledge for its function stored in the minds of the elderly men and women in the society, the youth of Africa are often seen as divorced from traditional values and hence are assumed to be the products of modern values. Contemporary African youth do represent a confluence of traditional African culture and Western modern values, but although they are constantly exposed to Western values through the media, their interpretations of these values are often based on their interactions with, and their relationships with, their families, and family relationships are often characterized by experiences that are based in traditional culture. Furthermore, young people may not fully understand or acknowledge the degree to which certain of their behaviors manifest their cultural experiences. Thus, the extent to which a young person acknowledges that his or her behaviors are grounded in traditional culture may be dependent on many factors, such as the opportunity for exposure to other cultural values, who the youth is communicating with and what the youth perceives that person to represent, and the culture of reference the youth believes that person represents.

Health Behaviors

Social responsibility, which includes responding strictly to family dictates, is still a major expectation most parents have of their children. This responsibility is an important reason parents screen the friends their children choose. As regards sexuality and preventing sexually transmitted diseases, youths are more likely than adults to be influenced by referent group normative values. Peer pressure to engage in high-risk sexual and drug-related behaviors may be more prominent in inner-city neighborhoods in Western countries, thus increasing the difficulty of communicating about AIDS (Morales, 1987). In the United States, for example, the images of African American males have been exaggerated such that stereotypical notions of sexuality have been internalized by young African American men (Davis & Cross, 1979; Wyatt, Strayer, & Lobitz, 1976). Appearing to be concerned about contracting HIV or using condoms during sexual intercourse may be inconsistent with this cultural norm. In fact, sanctions may be directed at those who attempt to engage in health-promoting behaviors (Fisher, 1988). Reference group identification and its resulting social influence may, therefore, be a powerful force in shaping behavior among African American youth. Thus, a peer-directed intervention may be useful in providing credible and positive role models and in creating a network of support to encourage the adoption and maintenance of self-protective behaviors.

However, youth are products of their environments, and they can be expected to behave in positive ways only as far as the support of adult guidance and their society makes possible. In this context, concern for sexuality decisions must be examined against such social mediators as unemployment and the relevance of the education and skills training youth receive to function in their society. Beyond these social concerns, there are social and cultural expectations that affect girls and boys differently. Young girls are faced with the pressure to experiment sexually just as boys are, but with the added burden of having to bear the brunt of the responsibility should an unwanted pregnancy result. Unwanted pregnancy is perhaps the single most important event that can take place in a young woman's life; it is certain to limit and can sometimes completely derail her prospects.

The pressure on young women to engage in sexual activity comes not only from young men but in many cases from older men who take advantage of the disadvantaged economic conditions of young women in their society to lure those women into sex. These men, often referred to as sugar daddies (*sour daddies* would be a more appropriate term), are responsible for significant numbers of teenage pregnancies in many African societies. The scenario is usually played out thus: A young woman is enticed with money to engage in sex with an older man and becomes pregnant; the man leaves, looking for other prey; the young woman withdraws from school or other activities that would have prepared her for a good future, and has her baby. Such cases happen all over the world, although they may be more pronounced in many Southern nations. Any policy designed to address the problems of youth in Africa must seek to criminalize the role these "sugar daddies" play in truncating the life possibilities of the women they exploit.

Using the PEN-3 method, we can identify positive, existential, and negative beliefs and practices associated with the health of young people. One positive area is the degree of curiosity found in youth and their willingness to learn, provided they are exposed to positive stimuli. An example of an existential practice is youths' reliance on adult figures for direction. An example of a negative belief is the common attitude among young people that they are immune to disease or injury.

Conclusion

If, as the Native American Indian adage says, "we have not inherited the land from our ancestors, we are borrowing it from our children," then we owe our children a great debt. Children and youth represent our future possibilities. To the extent that we fail them, we have failed ourselves. With so much emphasis on child survival, we must remember that it is also critical that we prepare our youth to make the smooth transition to adulthood.

The social and cultural production of youth in Africa places youth within the context of the family with certain responsibilities. Any discussion of the issue of youth is incomplete without special attention to the differential concerns of female youth, and the role older men play in perpetuating their marginal status. This concern is one that transcends geographic and regional boundaries.

NOW:

My conversation with Priscilla Madzinga-Kusena

Cultural and Professional Identities

Airhihenbuwa: see chapter 1

Madzinga-Kusena: Well, of course, I'm a mom, a wife, a daughter, an aunt, and lately, a grandma. My nieces and nephews have young children, so I find my roles shifting quickly. Culturally, there's so much to say, but I'll note that faith is also very central in the African setting. How we define ourselves often connects to how we align with God, through worship, giving time to church, and recognizing a higher being. Professionally, like you, I sit at an intersection. But in our field, it's becoming harder to clearly define our space. Public health now requires us to draw from many disciplines, economics, statistics, and digital innovations. It's no longer enough to just understand human behavior; now, competencies include financing and other skills. There's a lot of pressure, but so far, I'm managing and holding my ground.

Continuing Relevance of the Chapter

Airhihenbuwa: Do you think the chapter we're reflecting on is still relevant today, especially given your work with the African Union?

Madzinga-Kusena: Yes, absolutely. I teased out six key points that remain, in my view, timeless:

1. **Strong cultural lens on childhood and family.**
   As a mother of three, I see the enduring relevance of naming, kinship, and extended family. These remain central in African settings, even though Western contexts may approach family differently. These cultural anchors help us de-medicalize child health.

2. **Maternal role and child survival.**
   The chapter highlights the linkage between maternal well-

being and child survival. Even today, despite women participating in the workforce, our maternal role in child survival remains central.

3. **Programmatic challenges.**
   For example, immunization programs. While widely accepted under primary health care, they remain siloed and top-down, influenced by donor-driven approaches. The critique in the chapter is still true today.

4. **Youth versus adolescence.**
   This distinction made me laugh while reading, because the debate persists. The term "adolescent" medicalizes young people, while "youth" connects to social roles and identity in African contexts.

5. **Social norms and gendered risks.**
   Issues like older male partners in patriarchal societies, what we used to call "sugar daddies", still exist, though they manifest differently today. Women may have more choices now, but the phenomenon persists.

6. **Frameworks.**
   I found the PEN-3 model still very powerful in helping us identify what's positive, existential, or negative in culture, and in guiding interventions, especially for meaningful youth participation.

Expanding the Chapter for Today

Airhihenbuwa: How should we expand or reposition the chapter for the future?

Madzinga-Kusena: A few directions stand out:

- **Life-course immunization.**
  Previously, immunization focused on children under five. But what happens after that? We now need to emphasize immunization across the life span and link it to broader

models of primary health care, especially given donor withdrawal and financing gaps.

- **School as a platform.**
As a mother, I know how competing professional and caregiving roles intersect with children's education. Schools remain critical public health spaces, linked to water, sanitation, and hygiene. They should feature more prominently in the chapter.

- **Contextual differences.**
It's important to disaggregate across rural, peri-urban, and urban settings. Each has unique dynamics worth capturing.

- **Strengthening frameworks.**
We could couple PEN-3 with models like the Social Ecological Model or Social and Behavioral Drivers. This could help capture influences on maternal roles, youth decisions, and cultural dynamics more holistically.

- **Deepening gender and inclusion.**
We should address intersectionality, shared decision-making, male engagement, safe spaces for girls, and inclusion of young people with disabilities.

- **Implementation science.**
Adding an implementation framework, perhaps even a theory of change, would move the chapter beyond narrative into applied strategy.

On Youth, Donor Narratives, and Autonomy

Airhihenbuwa: You mentioned earlier the tension between using "youth" and "adolescent." Sometimes donors push the language of adolescence because that's where their funding is directed. How do you negotiate that tension?

Madzinga-Kusena: That's a real issue. At work, in my first week, we debated donor-driven narratives. Some donors dislike terms like "risk communication" or "community engagement" and push for their preferred terminology. When it comes to "adolescence" versus "youth," we meet them halfway. Officially, for donor-driven projects, we may use "adolescent." But in communities, we always use "youth," because that's the language people understand. Saying "adolescent" medicalizes young people and reduces their participation to tokenism. "Youth," on the other hand, resonates with community expectations and strengthens accountability. This balance allows us to satisfy donor requirements while keeping authenticity at the community level.

Schools, Culture, and Identity

Airhihenbuwa: You raised the point about schools earlier. How should lessons from the field be reflected in what young people are taught?

Madzinga-Kusena: Schools are crucial. Children now enter preschool as early as six months or a year. They spend most of their time in schools, so these spaces play a huge role in shaping identity, alongside academics. At home, we remind our children: *we send you to school for information, not identity*. Identity comes from culture and family. Still, schools influence culture, through peer-to-peer learning, cross-fertilization of ideas, and assimilation. So, while schools shape thinking, parents must provide checks and balances to preserve cultural identity.

Final Thoughts

Airhihenbuwa: Any final thoughts?

Madzinga-Kusena: Reading the chapter was like revisiting my childhood. It brought back memories and sparked conversations with my own children. They laughed, recognized examples from family life, and even said, "Wow, mom, this is good." That, to me, shows the chapter achieves its purpose. *It bridges generations,* *sparks dialogue, and grounds our identity in culture while pointing forward.* I look forward to this new edition of the book, and I hope this conversation helps shape it.

Chapter 7

Contextualizing the Health Praxis of African Americans

THEN:

> Unable to call upon the power of ancestors, because one does not know them; without an ideology of heritage, because one does not respect one's own prophets; the person is like an ant trying to move a large piece of garbage, only to find that it will not move.
>
> *Molefi K. Asante,* Afrocentricity, 1987

> You have to position yourself somewhere in order to say something at all. Thus, we cannot do without that sense of our own positioning that is connoted by the term ethnicity. And the relation that people of the world now have to their own past is, of course, part of the discovery of their own ethnicity. They need to honor the hidden histories from which they've not been taught to speak. They need to understand and revalue the traditions and inheritances of cultural expression and creativity. And in that sense, the past is not only a position from which to speak, but it is also an absolutely necessary resource in what one has to say.
>
> *Stuart Hall, Ethnicity: Identity and Difference, 1991*

Some professionals have suggested that there is no authentic African American culture, and therefore, alternative theories and perspectives on the health-seeking behaviors of African Americans are unnecessary. Some of those who do believe in the existence of an African American culture apparently view it as only a deviant variation of the majority culture (Aldous, 1969; Parker & Kleiner, 1969). Further, there are some who believe that even though there are some differences between African American culture and the dominant White culture, there is no value or benefit to be found in accentuating the differences without according equal coverage to other groups (West, 1993) - that is, confronting the issue of multiculturalism. However, there is strong evidence that African Americans stand to benefit more from health promotion and disease prevention programs when those programs are conducted in ways that affirm and legitimate African Americans' cultural codes and meanings. Such affirmation of differences in health promotion activities in African American communities should be promoted (Airhihenbuwa & Pineiro, 1988).

The project of legitimating and affirming the voices of African Americans' cultural space has been a focus of research and practice by scholars of African American culture. One example of this cultural project is Afrocentric theory, which is anchored in a belief in the centrality of Africanity in any analysis involving African culture and behavior. For instance, as Asante (1987) notes, "The communicationist who defines a speech as an uninterrupted spoken discourse demonstrates either a disregard or ignorance of the African tradition of speech, much as Leslie Fiedler showed a purely European conception of fiction when he contended that romance was a central theme in literature" (p.6). According to James Stewart (1992), Afrocentric theory tends to fall into two basic categories. The first is the

> `strong claim' - the assertion that the liberation of peoples of African descent requires a psychological reorientation that focuses on reconstructing selected aspects of traditional African psychology, values, and behaviors in the present. The second is the `weak claim' - the position that liberation requires that top priority be assigned to the interests of peoples of African descent in social and political intercourse with other collectives. (p.35)

African American cultural scholars have consistently challenged the application of traditional models based on White culture for recommending treatment and/or behavior change to promote health and prevent disease among African Americans. Research evidence confirms the lack of congruence of these practices with the

African American experience, lifestyle, and culture (Jackson, 1983b; Leonard & Jones, 1980). In response to these deficits, some researchers have proposed African- and African American-based personality and treatment models (Baldwin, 1981; Nobles, 1980; Parham & Helms, 1985). Consequently, new approaches for educational and behavioral change models have been advanced.

Afrocentric scholars tend to agree that African American values are a confluence of African heritage and the American experience (Jackson, 1983a; Nobles, 1980). Although the focus for many years has been on the American experience (Jackson, 1983a), scholars such as Asante (1983, 1987) emphasize retained African values and behavioral patterns. Examples include the extended family, the belief that all the aunts and uncles are responsible parents of all their nieces and nephews, the belief in collectivism as opposed to individualism, and respect for age (Allen, 1978). A lifestyle of acquiescence to nature rather than challenging it and an emphasis on oral tradition are also hallmarks of African values.

Jackson (1983b) notes: "Cultural theories in Black psychology are characterized generally by an emphasis on `wellness' or normality instead of psychopathology. The focus on normality in turn is based on an African value system" (p.20). Theoretical formulations are relevant only to the extent that cultural values are recognized and incorporated (E. T. Hall, 1977). Because health behaviors are culture-bound, primary prevention efforts that address preventable disease and illness must emerge from a knowledge and understanding of the target culture so that health interventions are culturally sensitive and linguistically appropriate (Braithwaite & Lythcott, 1989).

Stewart (1989) has called for the development and prioritizing of a grand theory of Africology based on a full understanding of the nature of history, time, space, and technology in Afrocentric terms. He argues that our political and intellectual efforts should be devoted to restructuring community ties and translating the language of African American intellectual elites into the language of African American popular culture. Such a framework will capture the beliefs of Africans and African Americans in postmodern history (Asante, 1987). However, some scholars, such as Marable (1993), have questioned the wisdom of analyzing African American culture and behavior based solely on African culture: “African, in effect, represents only one-half of the dialectical consciousness of African American people. Blacks are also legitimately Americans and, by our suffering, struggle, and culture, we have a destiny within this geographical and political space equal to or stronger than that of any white American” (p. 121). In the words of Angela Davis (1992), “There is no simple or unitary way to look at expressions of Black nationalism or essentialism in contemporary cultural forms” (p.320).

It is not my intent here to debate what constitutes the production of African American culture in the mid-1990s, but it is worth noting that even after African Americans' many years of lived experience in the United States, there still remain many compelling similarities between African Americans and Africans with regard to certain cultural codes and meanings in actions and behaviors. Such behaviors can be found in choices and values assigned to foods, the importance of orature and oracy in communication, and the use of traditional healing, all of which are important in the development of health promotion and disease prevention programs. In this context, this chapter focuses on the degree to which African Americans' health conditions can benefit from culturally appropriate paradigms that are grounded in historical correctness rather than mere political correctness.

In spite of efforts to understand cultural values as they relate to personal behaviors, little attention has been given to the development of a culturally appropriate paradigm for health promotion in the African American community. Currently, culturally sensitive educational and behavioral change models for health promotion in African American communities tend to be based primarily on the Caucasian experience. Attempts to make these programs culturally appropriate tend to rely on the individual and family psychology of African Americans. A major shortcoming of these models is the failure to ground personal crises in the social and political context within which the individual must function. It is critical to establish a balance between the behavior the individual can change and the social-political factors in the environment that must be managed before those changes are meaningful and sustainable. The outcome is that these approaches offer no models for translating known cultural and psychological realities into a working framework that could guide the development of culturally appropriate health promotion and disease prevention programs in African American communities. Myers and King (1983) present a dialectic crisis-conflict model for understanding mental health outcomes in the growth and development of the African American child. The uniqueness of this model is manifested in its recognition not only of the significance and depth of the personal crisis faced by the African American child but also of the etiological significance of the undeveloped consciousness in the victim of the fundamental social contradictions that he or she faces.

Given the faulty premise that African American culture is not different from White culture, it has been easy for Eurocentrists, health professionals, and laypeople alike to delude themselves into thinking that they are familiar with African American culture in all its aspects (Jackson, 1983a). The consequences of such a mindset include failed health care programs for African American communities - programs that may have been conceived out of genuine concern for the communities, but that have been methodologically and theoretically flawed. *There is no doubt that the failure to recognize the cultural inadequacies of conventional models, so as to train scholars and practitioners to use alternative cultural models, has contributed significantly to the profound disparity in health status between African Americans and the White population.* "The degree to which African Americans perceive the `odds against them' as manageable or overwhelming will depend to a significant degree on the transactional competency and success of their parents, the competence of the role models in their primary community of competency, and, finally, on the availability and accessibility of resources and supports to help them in their coping efforts" (Myers & King, 1983, p.20294).

Although socioeconomic status influences health outcomes, racial and cultural differences are also associated with the low health status of African Americans (Airhihenbuwa, 1989a). In the words of Derrick Bell (1992), "What we now call the `inner city' is, in fact, the American equivalent of South African homelands. Poverty is less the source than the status of men and women who, despised because of their race, seek refuge in self-rejection" (p. 4). Low economic status is linked with poor health status, and other factors, such as structural discrimination and institutional racism, favor the disproportionate representation of African Americans in low-income groups, which ultimately results in their poor health status. A focus on individual income fails to address the social context and environment in which a disproportionate number of African Americans find themselves (Auslander, Haire-Joshu, Houston, & Fisher, 1992). Even among African Americans whose income levels are the same as those of the majority White population, many other factors - such as total assets, housing, prior socioeconomic status, and social mobility - influence health status (Kumanyika & Golden, 1991).

A position paper adopted by the American Public Health Association's Governing Council in 1974 refers to racism as an established characteristic of the health care delivery system (cited in Muller, 1985). The impact of health service accessibility problems on African American families reflects the poor quality of care they receive. When choices for available services are limited or nonexistent, the quality of services is hardly ever questioned by public policy makers. The goal of the public health system in the United States should be the achievement of equity in the health status of all Americans. The discussion that follows examines some of the reasons gaps persist between the races in the delivery of health services.

Disparities in Health Status

Disparities in health status between African Americans and Whites have long been and continue to be realities in the United States. Blacks of both sexes and in all age groups are more likely than Whites to be ill or to die prematurely. The 1989 mortality data for Black men showed a continued reduction in life expectancy and no change for both sexes, in sharp contrast to the extension of life by 0.4 years for Whites of both sexes ("Health Trends,"1992). Age-specific excess deaths for Blacks compared with Whites in 1991 ranged from 64% for persons aged 15-25 to 11% for persons 65 years and older (Fingerhut & Makuc, 1992).

A Black baby is more than twice as likely as a White infant to die before his or her first birthday (Edelman, 1989). In 1989, the infant mortality rate for Whites was 8.2 per 1,000 live births, compared with 17.7 per 1,000 for Blacks ("Health Trends," 1992). The gap is even wider (8.1 for Whites and 18.6 for Blacks) when the mother's race is used to classify infant mortality rate. The proportion of low-birth-weight infants among Black mothers is almost three times that of Whites. The 1989 rate of 13.3% (compared with 5.7% for Whites) has been increasing yearly from 12.7% in 1980 (U.S. Department of Health and Human Services, 1991).

Effective use of available, accessible, and affordable preventive services can significantly improve maternal and child health. A major factor responsible for the disparity in health conditions of African Americans compared with Whites is the underrepresentation of African Americans as health providers. Proctor and Rosen (1981) found that African Americans may not always express racial preferences or expectations regarding their health care providers, but when they do, they indicate a desire to be seen by African American health care providers. Bonding along racial lines, even for an impersonal health care provider, suggests the strength of the historical experience of a group. To the extent that physicians rely on a patient's "will to live" as critical to the patient's prognosis, particularly after complicated surgery, the patient's "will to perceive" an acceptable health care provider is equally critical. Thus, we must take seriously the patient's assumptions about the competence of such a person on the basis of his or her racial identity and its compatibility with that of the patient. Even if an African American patient is not seen by an African American physician in a medical facility, the patient's knowledge of the presence of an African American practitioner in that facility can help to alleviate some apprehensions he or she may have about services. People who share similar cultural patterns, values, experiences, and problems are more likely to feel comfortable with and to understand each other (Levy, 1985).

Whitehead (1992) and others have proposed a cultural model (the cultural systems paradigm) designed to centralize culture in the understanding of the decisions and behaviors of African American individuals and families. This model has been useful for the conceptualization of a holistic approach to understanding culturally based food choices by African Americans. This model also takes into account the social, political, and environmental context within which individuals function.

The need to examine the personal or cultural health beliefs of African Americans is increasingly critical. For example, teenage pregnancy is an issue that has received increasing public attention in the past decade. In the development of health interventions targeting teen pregnancies, the assumption is usually made that all such pregnancies are unwanted. Consequently, interventions tend to concentrate on recommendations of birth control methods for all teenagers. Such recommendations, however, are totally irrelevant for teenagers whose pregnancies are planned, an increasing number of whom are African American. Programs aimed at preventing pregnancies among teenagers who want to become pregnant need to examine and address societal failures that condition these children to want to have children. Children having children is one concern, but children *wanting* to have children is another - there is no worse evidence that a society has failed its youth.

Dealing head-on with the truth of this individual construction of reality is not to suggest an endorsement of such reality, but to focus on the root causes of behavioral manifestations in human lived experience and growth. In other words, accepting the truth of some wanted pregnancies among teenagers can allow interventionists to explore why these teenagers want to have children. Both wanted and unwanted teenage pregnancies have important policy implications. Health and social practices are usually manifestations of several forces that collectively shape individuals' cultural beliefs and individual life experiences. In the case of children wanting to have and having children, the interventions that may be most successful in the long run may be those that concentrate on the systemic factors - such as failed government policies, high rates of unemployment, and various forms of marginalization and discrimination - that have contributed to teenagers' feeling that they have no other future.

Problems in Health Institutions

The notion of health care as a delivery system is a myth that continues to be perpetuated. The health care industry does not deliver health care, at least not to the African American community. The rendering of health care services (to those who can afford them) should be demystified and presented for what it is - a medical production. Once we understand that the health care system is a medical production, we can place it in relation to its political economy, that is, who produces it and how the producers control the costs of the services they render, who consumes them and how that consumption is rationed, and who has little access to services and why this is the case. Recent U.S. health care reform proposals have emphasized structural access as critical to ensuring universal coverage. Although this seems reasonable, it does not address issues of corporate/societal responsibility by way of, for example, criminalization of billboard advertising for alcohol and tobacco products that targets minority communities, enhancement of historically Black medical schools' ability to increase the supply of African American health providers, and promotion of cultural sensitivity among health providers and health programs that are central to providing meaningful universal health coverage to African Americans and other non-White populations. Concerns about access must not be restricted only to dollar costs for coverage of care; equally important are the opportunity, emotional, and spiritual costs of unacceptable services.

These latter costs are evident in research findings concerning the indices of availability, acceptability, and affordability, as well as accessibility, of health care services for African Americans. An examination of the availability of health care resources reveals that the condition has worsened for African Americans since the U.S. Department of Health and Human Services published its 1985 task force report on the status of Black and minority health (cited in Hale, 1992). Indeed, in a 1988 response to that report issued by the Commission on Minority Participation in Education and American Life, the investigators concluded that the United States is "moving backward" in its efforts to secure equity for minority citizens (Jacob, 1989). Reductions in federal financing programs slowed the decentralization of health care resources through block grants and attenuated the increasing accessibility of health care services for minorities and the disadvantaged. For example, the Health Education-Risk Reduction Grants Program was cut by 25% as a consequence of the 1980s block grant policy (Kreuter, 1992).

Even when services are available, they may not be as accessible to Blacks as to Whites, because Black families are often faced with different barriers that complicate their access to health services. For instance, some physicians refuse to treat patients who are indigent (Davidson, 1982) and some refuse patients who are Black (Charatz-Litt, 1992). Other barriers include limited access to medical facilities, long waiting times at medical facilities, inconvenient medical office hours, and the absence of privacy within public and private clinics and emergency rooms (Davidson, 1982).

The underrepresentation of Black professionals in the health care delivery system has complicated the problem of accessibility (Airhihenbuwa, 1989a). As of 1989, Blacks constituted 12.1% of the U.S. population, and 13.6% of the population aged 20 to 29, yet African Americans received only 5.3% of the medical degrees awarded in that year (Petersdorf, Turner, Nickens, & Ready, 1990). African

Americans accounted for only 5.8% of the total number of doctorates awarded in health education between 1980 and 1988 (Airhihenbuwa et al., 1989). Of the total number of graduates from schools of public health in the 1981-1982 academic year, only 2.5% were Blacks (Airhihenbuwa et al., 1989). As noted above, Proctor and Rosen (1981) found that when Blacks have a preference, they express a desire to be attended to by Black health care providers. African American counseling clients in Miles and McDavis's (1982) research expressed finding comfort in the knowledge that there were Black counselors on the counseling staff. An increase in the number of Black health professionals might well improve accessibility and subsequently the quality of health care delivery to Black clients. The presence of Black faculty in health education and other public health academic departments may directly or indirectly enhance the recruitment and, more importantly, the retention of Blacks in these programs (Airhihenbuwa et al., 1989).

Although increasing Black representation in the health care professions is important, of equal importance is an emphasis on cultural sensitivity among health care professionals. Medical schools and schools of public health need to offer courses that will prepare future health professionals to understand the differing cultural values and meanings of health and medical practice for their patients. Such education could be instrumental in breaking down the cycle of institutional racism. *Structural discrimination and institutional racism are synergistically responsible, in large part, for the persistent disparity between Blacks and Whites in the availability and accessibility of health services*. This is evident in the ways the policies and practices of the White medical community negatively affect the health of African Americans (Charatz-Litt, 1992) as well as in the history of racism as an established characteristic of the health care system (Muller, 1985).

Discriminatory practices in health care availability and accessibility are often exacerbated by the limited resources of many African Americans. Investigators have documented the disproportionate decrease in income levels among Blacks compared with Whites. Based on constant dollars, 30% more Blacks than Whites had an annual income of less than $5,000 in 1987 than had occurred in 1970 (Horton & Smith, 1990). Today, 34% of African Americans are below the poverty level, compared with 11% of Whites (Auslander et al., 1992). Opportunity costs, or the synergy of time and money required to access available health services, are also a major barrier to health care for the economically disadvantaged (Airhihenbuwa, 1992).

Services that are available, accessible, and affordable must also be acceptable to patients. Racism has separated Blacks and Whites to the extent that many White health care professionals are unaware of the Black experience (of suffering and discrimination, particularly) and the effect it has on Black people. This ignorance may prevent professionals from understanding both the cultural appropriateness of African American clients' behavior and the adaptive qualities of such behavior. White professionals may therefore discount the value of, or incorrectly label, the behavior of a Black client as abnormal. Conversely, ignorance of Black lifestyles may contribute to health care workers' tendency to attribute certain behaviors to racial differences when such behavior should be ascribed to personal malfunctioning and psychopathology.

Of the 10 leading causes of death in 1976, 50% were related to unhealthy behaviors or lifestyles, 20% to environmental factors, 20% to human ecological factors, and only 10% to inadequacies in health care (U.S. Surgeon General, 1979). Thus, doctors have little or no control over many of the factors that make us ill or keep us well. By focusing on lifestyles, social conditions, and the physical environment, health educators have been successful at improving the health of the population (Airhihenbuwa, 1989a). Because most Black clients receive care from White professionals, cultural differences often arise in doctor-patient relations. Many African Americans are suspicious of White health care institutions, at least in part because Blacks have historically been exploited for medical experimentation and demonstration (Jones, 1982; Pernick, 1985; Savitt, 1982).

Recent studies on health promotion and disease prevention have shown that improving self-esteem, building skills, and providing support are the three most important ways to promote positive health behavior change (Keeling, 1992). However, the improvement of self-esteem, building of skills, and provision of social support are all influenced by the degree to which individuals can influence other forces within their environments. The empowerment of individuals, groups, and communities rests upon their ability to understand and manage, or at least function adequately, within existing environmental forces. The next section explores strategies for promoting such abilities within the context of the African American family and community.

Health Promotion/Education Interventions

Existing health promotion strategies for U.S. ethnic minority populations tend to be based on theories and frameworks drawn from the White population. Although these theories provide insights into human behavior in general, they are inadequate for the planning, implementation, and evaluation of health promotion and disease prevention programs for African American communities.

Health promotion and disease prevention programs that target individual behavior change must not absolve the government of its responsibility to provide a secure environment in which individuals have the opportunities and resources they need to make decisions and engage in positive activities that lead to improved self-esteem. Bandura (1977) demonstrated that individuals' personal expectations of their ability to influence events in life (self-efficacy) determine whether they will initiate behavior to deal with particular situations, how much effort they will expend, and how long they will sustain the effort in the face of obstacles and aversive experiences. Those who believe they have the skills to cope will be more likely to use those skills if they have the resources to utilize them and the support and protection necessary to do so. Thus, skill development among African Americans is pivotal to their empowerment within the context of having the necessary supports and rewards from society.

Techniques used to facilitate the transition from powerlessness to empowerment among health care clients have embraced consciousness-raising, training in social competence that includes encouraging and accepting the client's definition of the problem, identifying and building upon existing strengths, analyzing how powerlessness is affecting the situation, identifying and using sources of power in the client's situation, the teaching of specific skills, mobilization of resources, and looking out for the client's welfare (Gutierrez, 1990). Another technique that should be developed is that of encouraging individuals and groups to work collectively toward changing negative policies and forces in their environments. The ideal modality for promoting empowerment is the small group, because it facilitates the use of such techniques as consciousness-raising, engaging in mutual aid, development of knowledge and skills, the modeling of behaviors, and problem-solving. Individuals in small groups can evaluate their effectiveness in influencing others and can receive support as they learn and practice new skills. Their interpersonal skills can influence their ability to influence others, to work toward changing institutions and social structures, and to attain personal and collective goals (Gutierrez, 1990; Ozer & Bandura, 1990; Saegert, 1989). This is true whether the goal is empowering individuals or institutions. Groups also provide support through the change process, a format for obtaining concrete assistance, and a potential power base for future action (Gutierrez, 1990). The outcomes of empowerment include changes at individual, interpersonal, institutional, community, and societal levels.

African Americans in different parts of the United States are assuming responsibility for finding solutions to the health and social problems that affect them and their families, despite the structural and psychological barriers that consign a disproportionate number of them to the lowest socioeconomic strata of society. The greatest contribution the government can make is to remove the barriers that frustrate the efforts of grassroots organizations to facilitate the empowerment of the African American family, because the latter remains one of the strongest institutions in Black communities. The African American family must become collaborators and solution co-creators before programs can effectively meet the needs of the Black population (Airhihenbuwa, 1989a).

Collectively and independently, African American family members must develop the skills necessary to lead to positive health behavior change. Health educators should partner with families to co-create the skills they need for collective efficacy and cultural empowerment. They can accomplish this by working with others in public health, particularly individuals of African descent (students as well as professionals), to identify and help address the needs of the community, as prioritized by the community. An example concerning food choices and food-related beliefs among African Americans, using the PEN-3 model, serves as an illustration. The application of the PEN-3 model allows health professionals to appreciate the social/environmental forces that may promote or threaten the success of positive health actions. Some positive health beliefs and actions among African Americans concerning food include the customs of eating green vegetables and eating at home with one's family. Existential health beliefs and actions include the drinking of pot liquor (the juice from cooked vegetables) and the belief that eating is a spiritual experience. Examples of negative beliefs and actions include the eating of greasy foods and reliance on fast food restaurants for daily consumption of unhealthy food.

While addressing individual behaviors, interventionists should also recognize environmental forces that may thwart individual efforts. An example of this is the availability of fast-food restaurants in most African American neighborhoods. This reality, coupled with the negative reinforcement of cigarette billboard advertising and liquor stores on every corner, represents forces that may require government intervention to control.

Preventive health initiatives can be introduced simultaneously with actions taken to address a community's prioritized needs, or after those needs have been addressed. *The Black Students Leadership Network, for example, combines community service with political activism.* This organization has worked to empower Blacks in housing projects to have control over the forces and decisions in their environment (e.g., influencing town council and community agencies' decisions about services provided in the community) that influence the destiny of their families and communities (Collison, 1992).

Sullivan (1989), a former U.S. Secretary of Health and Human Services, points out that one way to address the disproportionately high rates of infant deaths and deaths from chronic conditions among African Americans is through increased emphasis on health education and preventive care. This call for preventive strategies is appropriate and timely, but we must be cautious not to develop health promotion and disease prevention programs under the assumption that individuals have total control over the factors that influence their health. There is a tendency to believe that, given the right information and perhaps the right circumstances, individuals will be willing and able to change their health conditions. Indeed, largely as a result of health promotion programs, many Americans now engage in a variety of risk-reduction activities and, as a result, some have experienced improvement in, for example, lipid profiles, management of hypertension, and a decrease in obesity, as well as healthier cardiovascular systems (Sprafka, Burke, Folsom, & Hahn, 1989). However, placing so much of the responsibility for health promotion and disease prevention on the individual has serious limitations (Becker, 1986; Lamarine, 1989). As Becker (1986) observes, the focus on the individual "enables us to ignore the more difficult, but at least equally important problem of the social environment, which both creates some lifestyles and inhibits the initiation of others" (p.19).

The assumption that the distribution of information will result in changes in behavior assumes that the information is "correct" and/or unanimously acceptable. Yet the content of some health promotion messages can be misleading, or so confusing that individuals have difficulty sorting out the facts (e.g., the mixed messages we have received about caffeine in recent years). As Lamarine (1989) notes, the scientific bases of many recommended programs are not clearly established, and there is thus much misinformation distributed. For health promotion/education programs designed for African American communities the situation is even worse, particularly because environmental influences on health behavior (such as food deserts and food swamps) are often ignored.

Individuals gain the ability to navigate their unhealthy environments by acquiring the skills to review information critically and by raising their levels of consciousness through the support of and sharing with friends and families. They are then better able to make appropriate decisions regarding health-enhancing activities. The decision-making task is a serious challenge, because avoiding most preventable diseases requires individuals and families to make lifelong changes, and failure to make those changes rarely results in immediate illness. Consequently, individuals whose daily survival is a struggle may perceive limited benefit in adopting lifelong patterns that involve abstention, for example, from eating certain foods, engaging in unprotected sexual intercourse, smoking, or alcohol use. It is for the benefit of accentuating the connection between an individual's livelihood and positive health practices that African Americans must be empowered to develop the skills and support they need to make positive health decisions. For African Americans, support, either within community groups or in the larger society, is essential to the promotion of changes at individual and group levels.

Overall, individual and group empowerment of African Americans benefits all of society, because *African Americans who are empowered will have a greater sense of political efficacy*, a greater desire for control over their environment, greater civic-mindedness, and a general belief that success results from internal rather than external factors. These outcomes, in time, will result in positive contributions to the improved health status of African Americans. Even when people of color tend to be race-effacing in their cultural identities, their allegiance to their hitherto denied cultural heritages tends to become stronger in times of personal conflict and professional problems.

Cultural Factors in Promoting Health

Culture represents a set or sets of shared behaviors and ideas that are symbolic, systematic, cumulative, and transmitted from generation to generation (Nobles, 1985). Culture comprises a vast structure of language, customs, knowledge, ideas, and values that provides people with a general design for living and patterns for interpreting reality. As a way to clarify the dynamics of ethnic minority cultures, I offer the metaphor of the U.S. educational and health care systems as a salad bowl, rather than as the melting pot it has long been imagined to be (Airhihenbuwa & Pineiro, 1988). The melting pot concept assumes that every culture in the United States is assimilated into the mainstream White Anglo-Saxon Protestant culture, forsaking previous cultural identity and heritage in the pursuit of sameness. It is this melting pot mentality that leads health professionals to disregard cultural differences as critical factors that must be considered in the development of health interventions. Consequently, they employ what they believe to be culturally universal solutions.

The salad bowl concept recognizes cultural diversity and the separate and unequal statuses of different groups in U.S. society. If a nation's people all share common customs, origin, history, and language, then the United States could be considered a country of many nations, including African Americans, Hispanic Americans, Asian Americans, and Native Americans. The salad bowl concept approaches heterogeneity with positive rather than negative predisposition. Cultural differences affect health status and outcomes; therefore, health programs must be developed to address such differences. Understanding of the salad bowl concept is important for public health and health promotion because it is a necessarily prerequisite to the encouragement and development of culturally appropriate health programs.

HIV/AIDS Prevention Among African Americans

The prevention of HIV infection among African American women presents problems for health communication/education.

Behavior change strategies emphasize the use of condoms and spermicide, careful selection of partners, and abstention from sex. Programs attempt to provide women with the skills they need to negotiate with men for safer sex practices. Hankins (1990) argues that strategies based on empowering women to be more assertive in sexual negotiations are in themselves inadequate, because in both Northern and Southern countries, women "who are at higher risk for HIV acquisition do not have the power within sexual relationships to negotiate a change in the rules" (p.444). Black women in particular run the risk of being abused (Mays & Cochran, 1988) or of being rejected by men if they try to put these strategies into practice. For some women, the risk of losing a partner may outweigh that of contracting HIV.

The control of pediatric AIDS among African Americans is also difficult. For some women, childbearing is important to their sense of selfhood; an HIV-positive woman may thus want to take the 30-60% chance that her child might not be infected. Further, such a woman may not be able to obtain an abortion even if she wants one, because of her HIV status (Mitchell, 1988). The societal repression that has led to the powerlessness of many African American women, coupled with poverty and discrimination, has led to an apparent lack of official interest in the presence of HIV infection in women. Moreover, there is the exclusion of women from some treatment programs for drug abuse and for AIDS, and a lack of adequate maternity and other health services for women, resulting in a rather pessimistic view about the possibility of changing the risks of infection for these women (N. K. Bell, 1989; Hankins, 1990).

Doyle, Smith, and Hosokawa (1989) used individual counseling, group educational sessions, and various media (radio, newsletters, churches, and community social gatherings) to transmit a variety of health messages to African Americans. They found "churches to be the most effective means of reaching the target group" (p. 62). Direct face-to-face contact was also effective, particularly when the person making the contact was culturally and socioeconomically similar to the targeted individual. Lau, Quadrel, and Hartman (1990) have shown that parental influence on the health behavior of young adult children is greater than that of the children's peers. The use of contraceptives by African American girls has been found to be more strongly influenced by the involvement of their mothers than by that of the girls' peers (Nathanson & Becker, 1986).

The African American family's influence on children's health and the strengths of African American women should form the basis for health education programs for African American families. The PEN-3 model can be used as the framework for planning health interventions in African American communities. Program planners must identify positive, existential, and negative socioeconomic, health, cultural, and environmental factors affecting Black families and shaping the development and maintenance of their health-seeking behaviors. Barriers to behavior change must also be a part of this analysis. Community members (both women and men) and agencies must be involved in planning, implementing, and evaluating programs targeted to that community. To be effective, messages must be persuasive; care must be taken that they do not produce avoidance because of the fears they engender or because of their incompatibility with community group norms. Messages should address behaviors that individuals can change, and financial and other supports should be provided so that such change is possible.

Programs should be delivered by people who are credible to the community. This means that more African Americans must be recruited to become involved. Health messages must reach the people wherever they normally congregate: workplaces, homes, hair salons and barbershops, churches, bars, and streets. A concerted effort must be made to change the socioeconomic and other discriminatory health delivery practices affecting the African American family.

Conclusion and Recommendations

Health promotion programs have been effective in helping individuals to decrease their risks of some diseases, such as cancer, cardiovascular problems, and hypertension. However, targeting individuals for most health promotion and disease reduction efforts without considering the effects of their environments may be counterproductive, because few have control over most environmental factors that influence them. Interventionists must tackle the sociopolitical and environmental forces that influence health behavior within the context of the culture, utilizing source experts who can also serve as positive role models to influence behavior change (Airhihenbuwa, DiClemente, Wingood, & Lowe, 1992). Finally, to promote health-enhancing activities, all health professionals need to become advocates for the people for whom options are rapidly decreasing. For example, Illich, 1976, noted that the fact that doctors are available in greater numbers where certain diseases have become rare has little to do with the doctors' ability to control or eliminate disease. It simply means that doctors deploy themselves as they like, more so than other professionals, and that they tend to gather where the climate is healthy, where the water is clean, and where people are employed and can pay for their services (Illich, 1976, p.21). Health professionals need to focus on environmental and social factors that rob people of hope and dignity and that contribute to poverty and crime. If left unaddressed, these can become further contributors to the health risks of African Americans.

NOW:

My Conversation with Chandra L. Ford and Derek M. Griffith

Cultural and Professional Identities – Positionality

Airhihenbuwa: See my intro in chapter one

Ford: I identify first and foremost as a daughter, sister, auntie, and niece. My identity is deeply rooted in family relationships. I also strongly identify as African American, an identity tied to culture, power, race, and racism. I'm a Black feminist and activist. I am also a granddaughter. My maternal grandmother was a respected community mother, a "Miss Loretta", with an honorary doctorate and a powerful life story as a sharecropping refugee from the Deep South. She was fearless, refusing to tolerate disrespect, even at a time when many women were expected to wait for respect rather than demand it. Professionally, I struggle with reconciling my activism for racial justice within institutions with my academic role as a professor and research center director. Though I no longer work as a librarian, I still deeply identify with that professional foundation.

Griffith: I'm a son, brother, uncle, friend, and man of faith. A descendant of Jamaican and Guyanese immigrants, I identify as a Black man within racial and ethnic contexts. Much of my career has been about recognizing what others overlook, centering the margins. My parents, immigrants unfamiliar with the U.S. South, didn't know how to help me navigate racism. My early years in Omaha, Nebraska, near an Air Force base, and later formative years in Atlanta shaped this complexity.

Personal Journeys in Advancing Anti-Racism in Academia

Airhihenbuwa: In the book, I have a chapter on women's health, but there is nothing on men's health. Can you speak to your work and leadership in promoting men's health?

Griffith: My journey into men's health started by honoring those before me, people who lacked the language or ability to speak openly about what they endured. My father was one such person.

He was the second Black board-certified neurologist in Georgia and the first in Atlanta. Before that, he was among the first Black residents in the Harvard medical system. He once told the story of pulling into the hospital parking lot only to be told he didn't belong. Security was called to confirm his credentials. Instead of confrontation, he simply blocked access, no one would enter if he was denied. My focus on men's health emerged as I moved from psychology into public health, especially community-based health promotion for African Americans. Most programs lacked male participation. I began exploring masculinity and health, only to find few valid measures or research addressing this intersection. Our literature review showed a dearth of studies involving Black, Latino, or Asian men over age 40. No validated masculinity measures had significant relationships with health outcomes. That drove me toward qualitative work, to understand men's definitions of manhood, their aspirations, goals, and strengths. My approach became grounded in culture and context.

Airhihenbuwa: The last time I was in a classroom where Black men outnumbered others was during my undergrad years at Tennessee State University in the 1970s. Since then, as a department chair, a dean, and now a professor at Georgia State, I'm lucky to have even two Black men in a class of 20. We must stay committed to addressing structural harms against Black women and explore how similar structures imact Black men, without pitting them against one another. The focus should be systemic violence, not individual blame. Years ago, in *Ms.* Magazine, bell hooks wrote that women's liberation should not be a plantation where only women labor. That vision, of liberation that includes men, is part of what led to the concept of womanism. It's about connection and collective agency.

Ford: I see my public health work as a continuation of my family's legacy. Even as a child, I was drawn to health education, seatbelt campaigns, bicycle safety plans, and organizing fire drills. I believe something within me always called me to this path. Today, I walk in many worlds, including that of critical race theorists in law. While some critique public health dismissively, I approach it with love. I honor the sacred commitment of those in this field. My earliest personal encounter with racism was in college. Though fluent in German and having lived in Germany, my professor dismissed me on the first day because she assumed a Black student couldn't belong in her class. That experience sowed the seed for my career in studying racism and crafting strategies for antiracism. My work is informed by lived experiences, my own and others'.

Lessons from Civil Rights and Historical Struggles

Airhihenbuwa: We stand on the shoulders of giants. Now, we must pass the torch. Malcolm X and Martin Luther King Jr. had different strategies, one fostered critical consciousness, the other structural and systemic resistance. In Africa, this was also true of Steve Biko and Nelson Mandela. The future calls for grounded and contextual approaches. Anti-DEI backlash is shaking the equity tree. Tourists have left; now it's up to the residents to care for it.

Ford: My work is explicitly focused on racism. I try to build an intellectual movement across disciplines. Thank you, Collins Airhihenbuwa, for taking this journey with me. There's often a tension between framing through racism versus culture. As a Black feminist, I struggle with how elements of popular culture, like the N-word in gangster rap, are used in ways some defend as cultural, but that concerns me deeply.

Griffith: I remember our meeting at APHA in 2017 with leading scholars who may be considered the godparents of antiracism work. They charged us with maintaining the integrity of this mission as we edited APHA's first book on racism. It was a heavy, sacred charge. Many before us didn't have the chance to say the word "racism" in scientific spaces. Our work builds on their sacrifices. We must ask: Is your success contributing to health equity or merely self-serving? Are you part of a process or just focused on the product?

Teamwork and Intergenerational Collaboration to Promote Anti-Racism

Airhihenbuwa: There is a need for collaboration and community in academic and professional work. Individual success should not overshadow collective progress. Past scholars/leaders highlighted the value of "village-building" and working across generational lines to strengthen movements for equity. Intergenerational connection is essential. The elders we revere often didn't see themselves the way we see them now, they simply did what felt right and necessary. We built a village, and we continue to sustain it. That takes time and intentional effort, it doesn't happen overnight. In village-building, the question becomes: where is your village, and who is on the journey with you? Derrick Bell's *Confronting Authority* taught us that we fight injustice not because we know the outcome, but because we are committed to the process.

Griffith: This generation often doesn't recognize the sacrifices made by those who came before. We see the successes of past leaders but not the scars, the battles lost, the jobs forfeited, or the promotions missed. Their journey was not glamorous, it was costly. What I admire about both of you is how you honor those who came before you. What frustrates me is when newer scholars present ideas as if they originated them, without acknowledging the foundations laid before. *Innovation without lineage undermines our collective progress. We must teach that our work builds on layers, from the unseen roots to the visible structure.*

Ford: Sometimes, I just want to push past the "health equity tourists" and focus on what truly matters. I remember a problematic article published a decade ago in a major journal. I felt compelled to respond, but didn't have the time. Then, in the next issue, a collective response appeared, and I nearly cried with joy. It showed that we have a critical mass, scholars thinking deeply, using community data science, and making meaningful contributions. That's why we're seeing backlash, because real change is happening. And we must remember that not everything worth citing is in biomedical journals. Interdisciplinary work, from the humanities to the social sciences, has shaped this field. Young scholars need to understand that.

The Language of Resistance and Reimagining Health Equity

Airhihenbuwa: We're often being told that knowledge is neutral, disconnected from identity and experience. But our experiences shape what we observe and how we write. Growing up in Nigeria, we were punished for speaking our cultural language (Edo) in school, only English was allowed. Then I came to the U.S. and saw African American children discouraged from speaking Ebonics. Language connects race, culture, and identity.

Griffith: I've struggled with calls to change our language in the face of political resistance. Terms like "structural racism" were developed carefully, with scientific grounding. To abandon them now feels premature. Yes, we must be strategic about where we use them, grants may be restrictive, but academic journals still support us. The resistance shows that our language matters. It means something.

Ford: I identify as a feminist and womanist. My feminism was shaped in response to spaces where white women defined feminism in ways that sought to separate Black women from their families and communities. Our approach is more holistic, Afrocentric. We view ourselves as part of a collective. I've even considered developing a DEI project that includes only white participants, just to challenge current paradigms. There's also value in engaging those who are willing to "break the law of injustice." The African American community in the U.S. is now ethnically diverse. This diversity provides new ways of thinking, not just reframing old models but creating entirely new frameworks.

Training the Next Generation in Anti-Racism

Airhihenbuwa: For the future, I want to reiterate your earlier point, Griffith, about Malcolm X and Martin Luther King, Jr., and the importance of recognizing how their locations (South for MLK and North for X) matter in their political strategies. Geography shapes strategy.

Ford: I hope the next generation focuses on relationship-building and authenticity. You can't borrow someone else's soul. *Don't strive to be a "star", be part of a constellation. Stardom as a model is isolating and susceptible to exploitation by racial capitalism.* Think collectively. Also, be cautious of self-righteousness. You may work with people who aren't deeply committed to antiracism, but they still contribute. We shouldn't gatekeep based on rigid criteria. People evolve, and roles are fluid, we are not fixed as aggressor, victim, or bystander. Over the past 30 years, Black culture has been increasingly shaped, and distorted, by Hollywood. This harms us physically, mentally, and spiritually. It's time for culture and health to come together and raise consciousness. Black culture should be a vehicle for healing, not harm.

Griffith: Let me say something I haven't shared before. The attack on DEI might become a blessing in disguise. Federal funding has long restricted what we could say or do, especially if it involved activism or structural critique. But if those controls weaken, we may have new freedom to act boldly. We may finally be able to fund the work we've long dreamed of, unrestricted and community-driven.

Airhihenbuwa: A crown has been placed on racism. But now we can see it clearly, it's visible. We don't have to play games. We know who we're dealing with. I'm glad we're ending on that note. In Nigeria, growing up, cultural wealth wasn't valued like it is today. Now, I see cultural rootedness as a vital asset. Revisiting this chapter, I see my own wrestling with how to define Black culture, trying to honor its tensions. This is a powerful closure to a deeply meaningful conversation.

Final Thoughts

The conversation focused on both distinct and shared cultural and professional identities, and how these intersect with antiracism efforts to promote African American health and well-being. From a journey as an African American feminist and librarian, emphasizing the tension between personal values and academic roles, to work on men's health and masculinity, the discussion highlighted the need to address disparities impacting Black communities. Concerns included the underrepresentation of Black men in health fields and the importance of confronting structural barriers affecting both Black men and women. This conversation reinforced the urgency of continuing the fight against racism in academia and beyond. The work must be grounded in community, informed by history, and driven by a commitment to justice. Future scholars are called to prioritize collective well-being over personal acclaim and to remain steadfast, both humble and fearless, as they carry this work forward.

Chapter 8

Approaches to Health Promotion Beyond the Turn of the Century

THEN:

> To know who you are is the beginning of wisdom. By achievements, Africans are the people of the day before yesterday. In potential, we are the people of the day after tomorrow. In between, we have been a pawn in other people's desire.
>
> *Ali A. Mazrui*, The Africans: A Triple Heritage, 1986

Cultural imperialism is manifested in school curricula that hold up Western and European experiences as the only experiences of importance. Even when other histories, languages, and cultures are taught, the images and the instruments of learning are often designed such that they are rooted in the past; it seems that the achievements of other cultures are to be glorified only for their nostalgia value - they hold no future possibilities. There is often no attempt to connect any information about non-Western cultures with current political realities, power, and education. Persons who are the products of colonial/postcolonial realities are conditioned to believe that everything good about themselves and their cultures existed only in the past and should remain there (see Said, in Mariani & Crary, 1990). This has long been true for people of African descent all over the world, particularly in matters relating to health beliefs and practices.

The success of health promotion programs in Africa rests on the degree to which they are based on the sociocultural realities of Africans. "Economic and political control of a people can never be complete without cultural control, and here literal scholarly practice, irrespective of any individual interpretation and handling of the practice, fitted well the aim and the logic of the system as a whole" (Thiong'O, 1986, p.2093).

In a 1991 multiagency report on the future direction of health education, the International Union of Health Promotion and Education, the World Health Organization, and the U.S. Centers for Disease Control did not center on cultural issues as a critical element in the promotion of health. Some still believe that these issues ought simply to be acknowledged, not situated at the core of health promotion programs. At best, the agencies' report alludes to culture as one of several secondary factors to be considered in health promotion. This document fails to accent how culture informs the various domains and dimensions (personal, institutional, and societal) of health promotion. The absence of cultural appropriateness as a major theme in this important health education document is a terrible and unfortunate omission. *To flatten the relevance of culture as a commonsense issue is to reinscribe the notion of universal truth in health, education, communication, and development projects.* Common sense is not common; it is relative and shaped by cultural landscapes and locations.

Food, water, and air, in correlation with the level of sociopolitical equality and the cultural mechanisms that make it possible to keep a population stable, play decisive roles in determining how healthy adults feel and at what ages they tend to die (Illich, 1976, p. 20).

Health Education and Empowerment

Cultural empowerment in health promotion and education can be an effective tool that enriches the production and acquisition of knowledge for interventionists and their audiences. The emphasis on participation of people in group action and dialogue is critical to the extent that interventionists do not assume the population is powerless at both the micro and the macro levels of decision making. The process must not assume that the community lacks confidence in its ability to change the lives of its members. Participation as a tool for cultural empowerment is an important public health and health promotion approach that is an essential foundation for the kind of co-creation of learning that empowers both students/audiences and teachers/facilitators.

In order to realize fully the benefits of empowerment as a process that situates students/audiences as actors rather than factors, subjects rather than objects, and spectators rather than spectacles, cultural and educational theorists must examine and analyze the historical genealogy of classical pedagogy that disempowers the learner in a manner that Freire refers to as the "castration of curiosity" (in Freire & Faundez, 1989, p.35). Classical pedagogy places patriarchy, White and middle-class, at the center of discourse, and at the same time maintains Others - non-Western cultures, racial and ethnic minorities, women, and low socioeconomic classes - at the margin. *Ultimately, a pedagogy of culture is needed to centralize and affirm differences in cultural expressions, thus empowering learners to be actors and subjects in the production of knowledge and their social and cultural identity.* In this final chapter, I discuss the basic tenets of critical and border pedagogy, explore how this radical process informs health promotion within the context of culture, and discuss the need for health educators to promote diversity by centralizing hitherto marginalized groups in programs and curriculum development.

It has been argued that the preventive-medical model of health promotion/disease prevention efforts has a tendency to blame the victim, whereas the radical-political model may bias consciousness-raising efforts toward the interests of the health educators rather than those of the community. Under such a model, etic analysis is used when emic interpretation is not only customary but logical and empowering. In *Learning to Question* (Freire & Faundez, 1989), Freire relates an incident that took place in Mexico: An agronomist who was engaged in agricultural education through extension activities decided to help the Mexican peasants by proposing that the farmers replace their simple variety of maize with a hybrid variety to achieve greater yield in productivity. The farmers tried the hybrid successfully but subsequently changed back to their original maize variety. Had the agronomist engaged the farmers in the production and acquisition of taste, meaning, and pleasure in what was to be their new cultural reality, he would have learned, as he did later, that this simple variety of maize was grown for home consumption only and not for sale, as he had erroneously assumed. Most importantly, the farmers grew the simple variety of maize "to eat in their *tortillas* and the taste of the hybrid variety of maize was completely different from the other and thus represented a basic change in the culture of that community in the form of the taste of their *tortillas*" (p.93).

Another example comes from my experience as a health education consultant for USAID in Nigeria in 1990. As part of the community's income-generating activities, the farmers were encouraged to grow their yams with fertilizers for higher yield. They tried fertilizers successfully for a year, but then discontinued their use. The yams that were grown with fertilizers rotted after two months of storage, whereas the non-fertilized yams could be stored successfully for the six months that would elapse before the planting of yams in the new season. Yet another example is the distribution of oral rehydration solution packets, as described in Chapter 6. These packets eventually create dependency instead of empowering people (Werner, 1989), who should be taught to prepare their own solution using local ingredients and implements. "The `technical aid' conception of education `anesthetizes' the educatees and leaves them a-critical and naive in the face of the world" (Freire, 1973, p. 20152).

Empowerment in health promotion is often defined as "a process of helping people to assert control over the factors which affect their health" (Gibson, 1991, p.369). It has also been used synonymously with such indices as coping skills, mutual support, community organization, support systems, neighborhood participation, personal efficacy, competence, self-esteem, and self-sufficiency (Kieffer, 1984; Rappaport, 1981, 1984). This concept of empowerment evokes the notion that the control of environmental forces is the ultimate goal. Although this may be true, understanding those forces in order to initiate necessary transformations of reality is a legitimate outcome of empowerment. Thus, the objective changes resulting from empowerment are different because they reflect the varied needs of individuals, groups, organizations, and communities, and the contexts where empowerment occurs.

Empowerment should begin with educational institutions, so as to enlighten every student about the experiences and histories of diverse national and international communities (Airhihenbuwa & Lowe, 1994). Such institutionalization of empowerment is the hallmark of critical and border pedagogy.

Critical Pedagogy and Culture

Paulo Freire (1970, 1973) revolutionized pedagogical approaches more than 30 years ago by bringing to the fore the debate over European-centered versus multicultural pedagogy. Classical pedagogy disempowers students and audiences by, among other things, assuming that students can only acquire knowledge, not produce it. This pedagogical approach, or what Freire (1970) refers to as "banking education," totalizes the curriculum and pedagogical practices with White, male, Western culture at the center, while marginalizing diverse student cultures and histories (Giroux, 1992). The pedagogical manifestations of this monocentric all-or-nothing discourse have been challenged in cultural studies. Grossberg (1994) offers an alternative approach to cultural studies that is a confluence of hierarchical practice, which assumes the role of the all-knowing teacher; dialogic practice, which allows the silenced to speak; and praxical pedagogical practice, which offers people the skills they need to change their destiny. Grossberg's alternative approach rejects intellectual claims to authority even though the teacher does not have to abandon the position of authority.

In other words, the teacher/interventionist refuses to assume ahead of time that he or she has the appropriate knowledge, language, or skills; instead, he or she co-creates with people in a contextual practice in which he or she is willing to risk making connections, drawing lines, mapping articulations between different domains, discourses, and practices, to see what will work, both theoretically and practically. In fact, one could relate the three approaches in cultural studies to the three approaches in health education. The hierarchical approach in cultural studies is similar to the preventive-medical approach in health education; the dialogic approach in cultural studies is similar to the radical-political approach in health education; and the praxical pedagogical approach in cultural studies is similar to the empowerment model in health education. Finally, the alternative approach proposed by Grossberg is similar to the PEN-3 model I have proposed for grounding health concerns in cultural codes at both micro and macro levels of society. The connectedness between these alternative approaches is evident in the theoretical and practical symbiosis between cultural studies and health promotion.

Freire and Giroux, as well as other cultural critics and educational theorists, such as Hall and Jacques (1989), Illich (1976), Thiong'O (1986), hooks (1992), West (1993), Chinweizu (1987; Chinweizu, Jemie, & Madubuike, 1983), Minh-ha (1991), and Asante (1987), have challenged political, educational, and social systems that valorize the hegemony of White patriarchy of the Western culture while at the same time marginalizing women and people of other races and cultures. Border pedagogy and the discourse of difference must become central to pedagogical reformation (by this I mean the production of knowledge and social and cultural identity in schools, communities, and work sites, as well as domestic and international) in health and education. This rethinking of health and educational intervention approaches is particularly timely given the global currents of deconstruction (rejection of universal truth) of past existential boundaries and construction of new realities based on politics of representation (inclusive of health projects that represent diverse races, ethnicities, nationalities, and genders). Given the link between cultural expressions and health behaviors (Airhihenbuwa, 1993), it is critical that health education revisit the politics of its professional location in the world.

Crossing the boundaries of educational discourse, Henry Giroux (1992) deepens and transcends the possibilities of learning opportunities by inviting the engagement of students, audiences, and teachers in the production of knowledge, meaning, pleasure, and value. His critical analysis of the politics of possibilities (which he refers to as "border pedagogy", as they relate to education and democracy, informs a broader discourse of critical pedagogy. In his book *Border Crossings*, Giroux (1992) posits that culture is a foundation for pedagogical and political issues and thus must be central to schools' functions in the shaping of particular identities, values, and histories, by producing and legitimating specific cultural narratives and resources.

Border pedagogy points to the need for conditions that allow students to write, speak, and listen in a language in which meaning becomes multiaccentual and dispersed and resists permanent closure...border pedagogy offers the opportunity for students to engage the multiple references that constitute different cultural codes, experiences, and languages. (p. 28)

Although border crossing is advocated, it should be borne in mind that the border crosser is not a race-effacing agent. People of color cannot always assume White identity in terms of representation, as Whites can assume Black identity. Therefore, crossing borders may be subject to conditions of race, gender, and nationality, to mention but three.

A disciplinary engine that has been instrumental in propelling critical pedagogy to its current theoretical and practical state is cultural studies. For cultural studies, "the question of power must always be located in a field of struggle, not as a zero-sum game in which one either simply wins or loses, but, rather, as an ongoing effort to change the balance and organization of forces" (Grossberg, 1994). Thus, cultural studies seek to contextualize theoretical practice by rejecting the theory known in advance of practice as well as empiricism/practice without theory. "In reality, without theory, we lose ourselves in the middle of the road. But, on the other hand, without practice, we lose ourselves in the air. It is only through the contradictory, dialectical relationship of practice and theory that we can find ourselves and, if we lose ourselves sometimes, we will find ourselves again in the end" (Freire, 1993, p.132). The connection between cultural studies and health promotion and communication is evident in the linking of the best of practice with relevant theory, such that practice becomes a form of theorizing. In the domain of cultural identity advanced in Chapter 3 (the PEN-3 model), theorizing is manifest in practice.

Culture and Health Promotion

Health promotion programs must problematize and reappropriate empowerment processes to centralize cultural codes and meanings in ways that address how to harness existing power, which is not always evident as new ones are being tapped. Because the classical empowerment approach in health and education suggests a focus on individual actions instead of the transformation of institutional and social forces in the environment, the onus of behavioral change still tends to rest on individuals and families. Institutional and social forces that construct the production of health, education, and politics are still largely structured in a manner that oppresses and excludes the cultural and heuristic expressions of the marginalized. As Freire (1970) notes, "One of the characteristics of oppressive cultural action which is almost never perceived by the dedicated but naive professionals who are involved is the emphasis on a focalized view of problems rather than on seeing them as dimensions of a totality" (p.137).

In approaching the issue of oppressive cultural actions within the context of health education, I will not address the retrogressive posture of neoconservatives regarding their own educational and political project, which consistently promotes Eurocentrism as universal truth. According to Giroux (1992), "The neoconservative agenda for higher education includes a call to remake higher education as an academic beachhead for defending and limiting the curriculum to a narrowly defined patriarchal, Eurocentric version of the Western tradition and return to the old transmission model of teaching" (p. 93). Moreover, 'Black conservatives focus on the issue of self-respect as if it were the one key that would open all doors to Black progress. They illustrate the fallacy of trying to open all doors with one key: they wind up closing their eyes to all doors except the one the key fits" (West, 1993, p.66). Rather, I will use critical analysis of the shortcomings of the liberal agenda to inform the future direction of health education. In the words of Giroux (1992):

> Dominant strains of liberal ideology have fashioned their anti-racist discourses on a Eurocentric notion of society that subordinates the discourse of ethics and politics to the rule of the market...it is precisely this assumption that prevents them [liberals] from questioning how they, as a dominant group, actually benefit from racist ideologies and social relations, even as they allegedly contest such practices. (p.115)

Herein lies the challenge faced by health educators, particularly those of us who have been told on more than one occasion that socioeconomic status is solely responsible for the disparities in health outcomes between Caucasians and people of African descent. Such a reduction of health disparities to class or social formation totally undermines the incongruence between the construction of learning opportunities in the schools and the cultural expressions of the Others, whose experiences are not central to the model of learning in the schools.

> Neither sociologists nor journalists have shown much interest in depicting poor whites as a "class." In large measure, the reason is racial. For whites, poverty tends to be viewed as atypical or accidental. Among Blacks, it comes close to being seen as a natural outgrowth of their history and culture. At times, it almost appears as if white poverty must be covered up, lest it blemish the reputation of the dominant race. (Hacker, 1992, p.100)

Central to this debate in health promotion is the need to challenge classical pedagogy that continues to valorize the White middle-class male culture while relegating Others to the status of voyeurs. A new politics of representation must be constructed to create a space in which different voices are heard and legitimized. "The new cultural politics of difference shuns narrow particularisms, parochialisms, separatisms, just as it rejects false universalisms and homogeneous totalisms" (West, 1990, p.34). Approaches to public health, health promotion, and communication should be reformulated so that pedagogical experiences centralize and affirm the experiences of the Others, whose historical and cultural experiences have hitherto been on the margins of their learning experiences. Attempts to promote cultural differences in schools and communities often manifest themselves in calls for program and/or curriculum integration, although program/curriculum reformation is a more progressive approach to centralizing diversity in the learning process. In some cases, special programs are developed to redress the grievances of the marginalized. In the United States, attempts are often made to atone for racism through measures aimed at eliminating racist institutional barriers in the marketplace and at providing compensatory programs to enhance the cultural capital and skills of African Americans, as are evident in various remedial programs in education and the workplace (Giroux, 1992).

Although the elimination of institutional barriers ought to be considered in programmatic efforts, the primary tool for exclusion often lies in the Eurocentric model of learning employed in schools. For example, in contrast to the Eurocentric model, Barbara Christian (1987) has observed that African American people have always theorized in narrative forms, "in the stories we create, in riddles and proverbs, in the play with language, since dynamic rather than fixed ideas seem more to our liking" (p.52; quoted in Giroux, 1992, p. 131). I do not mean to assert here that all African Americans are alike in their production and acquisition of knowledge, but rather to argue for the legitimation of one valued form of cultural production found among African Americans. The differences in production and acquisition of knowledge and values of many African American children are not central to school curricula. Jacqueline Jordan Irvine (1990) writes:

> White middle-class parents and white middle-class teachers used "known-answer" questions, which solicited responses to names, shapes, and colors of objects. On the other hand, the Black children and their parents engaged in more sophisticated verbal storytelling involving the use of metaphors and analogies. In school, Black children asked questions such as "What's that

like?" or "Who's he acting like?" rather than the more middle-class attributional "What's that?" (p.23)

Professor Asa Hilliard of Georgia State University has found that White children tend to tell stories in a *linear* fashion, whereas African American children are more apt to employ a *spiral* style, similar to learning styles found in many African cultures. When given an assignment, they frequently "skip around to several apparently irrelevant topics before they come back to the theme, and then they begin to work on it" (cited in Hacker, 1992, p.172).

Educational reforms that focus on legitimizing cultural differences have important implications for research methods. "The general method of oral history research has appeal to Black/Africana Studies because of the importance of oral communication in the historical experiences of peoples of African descent" (Stewart, 1992, p. 2015). Such a focus on the significance of orature in research methods does not compromise the value of other hitherto exalted research methods; rather, it deepens and extends the possibilities for understanding cultural productions among people of African descent. African Americans, for example, must construct multivalent and multidimensional responses that articulate the complexity and diversity of their practices in the modern and postmodern world (West, 1990). If diversity is not central to the construction of learning opportunities in U.S. schools, the reality for African countries is even more troubling. The fixation on seeking so-called universal truths (the melting pot mentality) has negatively influenced the learning possibilities that legitimate and affirm different cultural meanings (the salad bowl paradigm) (Airhihenbuwa & Pineiro, 1988). The result has been the development and implementation of health programs that fail to recognize and centralize cultural influences of health practices and behavior.

Conclusion

The future of health promotion and disease prevention strategies as components of the operationalization of health, education, and development goals lies in the ability to centralize the discourse on culture and the politics of representation at the core of programmatic and philosophical enterprise. Such a process should include the inscription of culture at the core of preventive health programs, at the same time they draw on cultural studies, philosophy, education, and the traditional disciplines of influence, such as medicine and sociology, to retheorize and reconstruct health education. Grounding a health promotion episteme in the ideologies and concepts advanced in critical/border pedagogy will be a step in the right direction.

A pedagogy of culture should become central to health promotion intervention strategies in a manner that does not naturally couple the concept of barriers with cultural differences. Programmatic efforts should deepen the possibilities of critical pedagogy as a part of health promotion practices in schools, communities, and work sites, as well as at national and international levels.

NOW:

My conversation with Caroline Kingori, Mienah Z. Sharif, and Khadijah Ameen

Cultural and Professional Identities

Kingori: I come from a very large family scattered across the globe. I am a grandchild of our late grandfather, who was the Senior Chief of the local town, a community leader known for initiatives that still define our local town today. I am a daughter, a sister to two siblings, and part of a broader extended family, where cousins are siblings. I enjoy traveling, cooking, music, time with family and friends, and supporting community engagement and advocacy. Professionally, I am a professor of community and public health, an administrator, a public health podcaster, and a co-owner of a women- and family-owned coffee business.

Sharif: I appreciated the way the identity question was framed; it allowed us to move beyond institutional affiliations. I no longer introduce myself by my job title or university; I say I receive a monthly deposit from X University, highlighting how conditioned we are to professional identifiers. Personally, I identify as a child of the Afghan diaspora. I was born in Germany to Afghan refugees and raised between Germany and the U.S. Because of this, the notion of home is constantly evolving. As someone with refugee lineage, I believe that a sense of "home" or "belonging" is a privilege denied to many by the very systems that created displacement. I reject the idea that anyone is voiceless; rather, I use my privileges to amplify voices made to feel voiceless. My affiliation is not geographic nor bound to a professional title, my allegiance is to people around the world committed to collective liberation.

Ameen: I am a daughter of the African diaspora, with deep ties to Black communities globally and in the U.S. South, where I was raised. I'm grounded in the long-standing traditions of Black Southern liberation practices. Professionally, I am a community-based social scientist and public health practitioner who engages in transdisciplinary methods across public health, anthropology, the social sciences, and the humanities. I am guided by a Black feminist paradigm. When I read the chapter, I read it through this lens. I also identify as someone with a hybrid role, a scholar-activist. My work, research, teaching, and service, are aimed at informing social action and aligning with community-based social justice.

Relevance of Social Justice in Public Health

Airhihenbuwa: When this book was written 30 years ago, I could say, perhaps, it was written for the three of you, and the educational contexts in which you found yourselves in your training. Now, 30 years later, when you think about the students you are training for the future, *is this chapter still relevant*? If so, in what ways would you add and/or expand today as you are engaged with training of the future generation?

Sharif: *My first thought while reading the chapter was: "Where was this when I was in school?"* These ideas weren't part of the dominant discourse, certainly not central to traditional public health curricula. You'd have to seek them out as part of a specialization. That has always troubled me. I've continued to grapple with those gaps and push against dominant paradigms even though I'm considered early-career. My principles and non-linear path delayed my entry into academia, I questioned then, and still do, whether it was the right direction for me.

To answer your question, *yes, it's absolutely still relevant. In fact, it may be even more so now.* In recent years, terms like "anti-racism" and "decolonization" have gained popularity but are often co-opted and diluted. That's dangerous. I think we need to critically interrogate and challenge the very systems we're part of. Otherwise, we're left with symbolic gestures that serve interest convergence rather than actual transformation. They reinforce systems of power and leave structural oppression intact.

What would you add to the Chapter Today?

Sharif: What would I add to the chapter? Not so much add, but I would say it already gives voice to the structural factors that remain absent in mainstream training. Even when public health discusses social determinants of health, the focus is often reduced to interventions at the individual or interpersonal level. What's missing in many curricula is a truly global or international lens. I personally avoid using the term "global health" because it reifies colonial paradigms, it's Eurocentric and American-centric. Global health is often just shorthand for the Global South, creating an artificial bifurcation between the so-called Global North. For me, public health is public health, full stop. I pursued my doctorate with a focus on climate refugees and food security. I was told I didn't belong in community health sciences and was pushed toward global health departments. But I chose community health because it allowed me to use an international lens to study immigrants and refugees in the U.S. Still, I encountered attempts to indoctrinate me with outdated theories like acculturation, concepts that ignore lived experience.

In terms of what I'd add to the chapter, I'd emphasize that the examples you gave, particularly from African contexts, also resonate with me deeply. These dynamics aren't unique to Africa; they apply across the Global South. Cultures in these regions are often seen as inferior, exotic, or, in the case of Muslim communities (or communities racialized as such), even inherently violent. That framing is harmful and inaccurate. It reminds me of another problematic concept in public health: the "intervention." The idea that we are intervening on a population implies superiority, that we are coming in to fix or improve a situation. But as we all know, those interventions often don't lead to the outcomes we claim. In fact, I think the field itself needs to be intervened upon. That's why Public Health Critical Race Praxis (see related reference) is so important, it encourages us to challenge not just our subjects but our own discipline.

Global Interconnectivity in Disciplines and Practices

Airhihenbuwa: As you read the chapter, you may have noticed references to cultural studies, which held significant academic currency at the time. It represented a convergence of work in the humanities, health, and social sciences. Communication studies, in particular, was pushing boundaries and had a big influence on my thinking. Paulo Freire was foundational, as were several African scholars. I'm curious, today, what body of work or area of thought would you say functions in a similar way for your own work?...

Ameen: The first thing that comes to mind is how public health, and really the social sciences more broadly, often privileges research capital over teaching and pedagogy. This chapter does a great job of bridging that divide. Today, I believe we need to center critical, cultural, liberatory pedagogies, both inside and outside the classroom, as vehicles for justice. I once took a liberatory pedagogy course in the College of Education, and I saw clear overlaps with Black feminist and critical cultural traditions. These offer powerful frameworks for rethinking the classroom as a site of liberation. But that vision clashes with the realities of academia. There's a real tension between pedagogical possibilities and institutional demands. Also, let's be honest, there are structural forces that pose serious challenges to critical scholars. These include public health accreditation bodies, major funders, and university systems themselves. They often limit how much resistance faculty, students, and staff can offer without risking their careers.

Airhihenbuwa: Yes, exactly, the question becomes: How do we transform the hegemonic gaze while still operating within its institutional lenses? Some critical scholars argue that if certain funding sources were to disappear, a potential benefit could be the ability to speak more freely. These funding structures often shape what we can and cannot say. And on the subject of liberatory pedagogy, there's a lot we can learn from theology, especially from traditions in Latin America and among Black theologians in the U.S. They've challenged how organized religion can erase identities and enforce hierarchies through moral and ethical codes. There are parallels in how pedagogy can be deployed to resist or challenge oppression.

Kingori: The chapter is already quite comprehensive. For me, public health is inherently interdisciplinary. We've always drawn from different fields, especially community engagement and alternative medicine. I believe we need to continue incorporating these perspectives into the classroom. Personally, I've always been drawn to medical anthropology, it brings together so many aspects of health issues that are relevant to our work.

Airhihenbuwa: The foundations of what we now call intersectionality, equity, and inclusion are rooted in critical race theory (CRT). Although CRT emerged from legal scholarship, it wasn't limited to law. Its aim was to expose how systems, not just individual bad actors, produce and sustain inequity. It helps shift our lens from isolated incidents to structural forces. Understanding what Derrick Bell and Kimberlé Crenshaw were advocating is essential for anyone working in this space. Even though CRT has been distorted in the public discourse, its original intent remains powerful.

Sharif: I want to thank my colleagues for everything they've shared so far, and thank you for these questions, they create space for a conversation we rarely get to have. As for culture in public health, I feel the field is profoundly lazy in how it engages with it. I don't think culture is ambiguous or unknowable. I think calling it that is a form of intellectual laziness, an unwillingness to learn, to appreciate different ways of knowing and living. The phrase "cultural difference" has become a convenient excuse to not engage. That, to me, is a manifestation of white supremacy. It says, "I don't need to understand you because you're already too different, too complicated."

Public health as a field is largely ahistorical. This absence helps perpetuate cultural erasure and othering. It disconnects us from the structural and historical forces shaping health. Yet, our struggles are interconnected, and so are our strategies for liberation. These silos we create only obfuscate that truth. I see myself as a child of global communities. I see only connections, whether it's mass incarceration in the U.S., the War on Terror in the Middle East and Africa, or the multiple genocides we are witnessing now across spaces. These are linked. I loved how the chapter opens with cultural imperialism, naming the U.S. and Europe as empires. Public health is inherently political. And we must explicitly challenge its apolitical stance in training programs and commonly used frameworks.

Your opening question about integrating the personal and professional was so powerful. But academia rarely values that integration. When we build authentic relationships with communities, we're reminded of the importance of humility, and of how complicit we are, at times, in the very systems we seek to critique. At the end of the day, I talk about structural oppression, yet a university paycheck pays my rent. My self-reflexivity includes acknowledging that tension. It also reminds me of how, in graduate school, I was shocked that the public health curriculum didn't require a course on international relations. This goes back to how "global health" gets artificially separated. Racism impacts health globally, but many schools don't even offer a class on war and health, unless it's an elective. If we studied imperialism and structural violence properly, we wouldn't need separate courses on immigrant or refugee health. The root causes would already be understood.

And finally, I think we must challenge the field's obsession with prioritizing quantitative methods. Storytelling, qualitative inquiry, these are often marginalized, yet they offer deep insights. Why are we so afraid to just listen? Why is that not enough? When I read your chapter, I kept thinking of bell hooks, particularly her writings on democratic education. I reread her work before every course I teach. She envisioned the classroom as a space for building community and raising critical consciousness. That aligns deeply with your critique of the banking model of education. Ultimately, it's about exposing and resisting systems of power, starting right in our own classrooms.

Advancing Liberatory Goals in Academia

Airhihenbuwa: This has been such a culturally replenishing exchange. You've each shared insights that deeply resonate with the traditions I drew on when writing this chapter, particularly African structural thought and relational dynamics, even in matters like road design. These structures are not just physical; they represent a logic of interdependence.

Kingori: I want to close with a question that's been weighing on me: What does "public" really mean anymore in public health or public education? Currently, there is a trend encouraging students to report their professors, which raises important concerns about academic freedom and the dynamics within educational institutions. This chapter addresses the concept of liberation; however, many individuals within the system may feel constrained. There is a longstanding perception that educational institutions can, in some ways, influence or manipulate thought processes. This creates a sense of conflict for many educators and students alike. While there is a desire to support a liberatory vision in education, practical challenges often hinder its realization. The financial realities of needing a stable income can further complicate the ability to advocate for change. The ongoing struggle lies in reconciling these aspirations with the actual practices within the educational system.

Ameen: I deeply echo that sense of conflict. As I finished my doctoral program, I was grappling with the same tension. And I want to lift up something else: your work, Airhihenbuwa, with the PEN-3 cultural model and public health critical race praxis shows how critical epistemologies, whether cultural, decolonial, or feminist, can inform how we teach and how we engage with students and communities. *We need to emphasize co-construction of meaning in the classroom*. We must move away from hierarchies where instructors are the sole knowledge-holders. Dialogue, storytelling, and art-based approaches, including community-driven knowledge generation, must be part of how we teach and engage. These methods honor lived experience as a legitimate source of knowledge.

Sharif: Thank you for this space. So much of what was said resonates deeply with me. I've been grappling with many of the same tensions and contradictions, and I want to close with a question I ask myself every day: Are these liberatory goals and values we hold even possible within the systems we work in? You laid it out clearly in the chapter; these tensions are not new. That's why having a historical perspective is essential. The systems we're trying to change are the same ones that commodify anti-racism today. I was formally trained to work in international humanitarian aid. But it wasn't until I went to Afghanistan and later studied international law and development in London that I encountered a critical view of humanitarian aid agencies and learned about the non-profit industrial complex. There, I was asked: Do you think our dominant humanitarian aid apparatus is even designed to see these post-conflict contexts be "developed" sustainably and sovereignly? Fast forward 20 years, and I now ask a similar question of public health: Do we really want to eliminate health inequities? Because if we did, what would happen to our jobs and the lucrative enterprise that is "health disparities" work? We must interrogate the commodification of this work, whether it's culture, anti-racism, or equity. How much money has been spent on "cultural competence" or "diversity training," and what has it yielded? We need a systematic review of how culture has been operationalized in public health, and what it has truly accomplished.

Airhihenbuwa: Those are exactly the right questions to ask. And asking them is itself part of the work, part of our collective self-reflexivity. When I speak about this journey, I sometimes reference Albert Camus's reinterpretation of the Greek myth of Sisyphus. Traditionally, Sisyphus's plight was considered a failure, repeatedly pushing a boulder up the hill only to have it roll back down. But for Camus, the act of continuing despite knowing the outcome is futile was itself a form of triumph. Likewise, Derrick Bell's work in critical race theory reminds us: we engage not because we are assured of success, but because we are committed to the process. That commitment is also at the core of Paulo Freire's philosophy, his idea of being in exile in one's own home, and Theodore Adorno's notion that “the highest form of morality is not to feel at home in one’s own home.” These thought leaders and their values helped shape my personal mantra, which became my tagline at Penn State in the 1980s: “Be comfortable with being uncomfortable.”

Final Thoughts

Overall, we shared diverse perspectives from different cultural backgrounds and professional roles, covering experiences and insights about public health education, cultural identity, and the politics of engagement. We explored ways to expand public health to include critical cultural perspectives and liberatory pedagogies, while acknowledging the challenges of implementing such approaches within existing academic and political systems. We discussed the importance of continuing to engage in the work despite uncertain outcomes, drawing on philosophical ideas about discomfort and self-reflection. We pointed to the importance of maintaining historical perspective and connections with past efforts. My final message was that we must be like the anthills Chinua Achebe wrote about in Anthills of the Savannah, bearing witness to the devastation of the past in the form of preserving the memory of what was left after the fire, lest the new grass grow unaware. The anthill may look barren to the untrained eye, but it holds stories of survival and continuity. Without it, the new grass might believe it is the first and the beginning, disconnected from what came before. We live in a world where ideological fires are blazing and threatening to erase our cultural and professional landscapes. But there is deep value in staying committed, even when the outcome is uncertain. Yes, *Be comfortable with Being Uncomfortable!*

Conclusion

THEN:

> Cultural hegemony is never about pure victory or pure domination...it is never a zero sum cultural game; it is always about shifting the balance of power in the relations of culture; it is always about changing the dispositions and the configurations of cultural power, not getting out of it. There is a kind of "nothing ever changes, the system always wins" attitude, which I read as the cynical protective shell that, I am sorry to say, American cultural critics frequently wear, a shell that sometimes prevents them from developing cultural strategies that can make a difference. It is as if, in order to protect themselves against the occasional defeat, they have to pretend they can see right through everything - and it's just the same as it always was.
>
> *Stuart Hall, "What Is This `Black' in Black Popular Culture?"* 1992

Emerging critical discourses of feminism, postmodernism, and postcolonialism have been successful in remapping the terrain of progressive theoretical discourses. These discourses have been successful neither in recognizing the importance of pedagogy as a political project (Giroux, 1994a) nor in accenting health as cultural production in the politics of representation. What I have attempted in this book is to accent culture within the context of health as one insurgent strand in these discourses. Thus, it was necessary for me to challenge existing public health assumptions and models by decentering traditional views of health, communication, education, and development and inserting the formerly omitted element of culture into their theories and practices. No critical educator, theorist, or behavioral or social scientist can afford to ignore the relationship of health to culture and vice versa.

As I have noted in the preceding chapters, a major requirement in engaging a healthy culture project is that we move beyond the decolonization of classical paradigms and the decolonization of present Eurocentric and patriarchal professional practices. "Decolonization often means de-westernization as taught by the White man. The latter continues to arrogate the right to tell the previously colonized how to unshackle themselves, and to pronounce whether so and so has successfully returned to his or her own kind" (Minh-ha, 1991, p.20). Decolonization is a cleansing enterprise that must be engaged by both the colonizers and the colonized. Although attempts have been made to problematize the hegemonic tools of oppression that privilege the West and patriarchy, it is equally important that the oppressed critically interrogate their position so as to expunge from their minds theories and practices that are embedded in a colonial mentality. "The decolonization of the African mind must therefore be seen as a collective enterprise, as a communal exorcism through an intellectual bath in which we need one another's help to scrub those nooks of our minds which we cannot scrub by ourselves" (Chinweizu, 1987, p. 9). Equally as important as decolonizing the minds of the marginalized is decolonizing the minds of the colonial masters. Scholarship that explores the minds, imaginations, and behaviors of the oppressed is valuable, but equally valuable is a serious intellectual effort to examine what racial ideology does to the minds, imaginations, and behaviors of oppressors (Morrison, 1992). Understanding the psychosocial functions of the role of racism in the minds of the oppressors is critical to the development and planning, for example, of cultural sensitivity workshops that should benefit the dominant population. By emphasizing the importance of the unconscious and questioning the validity of a universal subject as the center of signification, Africans are demanding a new understanding of the human sciences and a redefinition of anthropology, history, and psychoanalysis (Mudimbe, 1988).

> This process challenges the oppressed to become engaged in politicizing and constructing health, communication, education, and "development" projects for the production of knowledge and codes that are consistent with their cultural meanings. It also demands that the privileged ideology must understand and affirm the importance and "seriousness" of the scholarly projects of the Others who engage in linking the political with the practical as a

> theorizing enterprise. According to Derrick Bell (1992), in the United States, ethnic minority educators whose research is oriented toward political or practical issues are often dismissed as having introduced ideological concerns into scholarship. As a result, the selection process favors Blacks who reject or minimize their Blackness, exhibit little empathy for or interest in Black students, and express views on racial issues far removed from positions held by most Blacks including - often enough - the student groups who urge the hiring of more minority teachers. (p.140)

Politics and education must be understood in their symbiotic roles in the production, distribution, and acquisition of knowledge. Excising the political from the life of the mind is analogous to a trembling hypochondriac always insisting on undergoing unnecessary surgery in spite of the sacrifice and high cost (Morrison, 1992). If politics is educational and education is political, outcomes should be measured by the extent to which politics and education equate culture-specific and culture-relevant health status with transformative and historical possibilities.

The affirmation of "Otherness" invoked in the politics of representation also underscores a recognition that Others are torchbearers whose political and educational projects often lead to the discovery of new truths as well as the affirmation of old truths. Quite often, when writers of oppressed races and nationalities insist that all writing is political, the claim has been dismissed as foolish or simply ignored, but when the claim is made by European philosophers, it is taken up as a new and original "truth" (Alcoff, 1991-1992). On a similar plane, the unimodal analysis of Western culture for universal applications has misguided scholars into concluding that if a person's work appears similar in style and theme to previous work, he or she must have been influenced by such "Western" work. Although this may sometimes be the case, it does not hold true within the context of multiple truths.

As Chinweizu (1987) has aptly observed, just because I am older than you does not mean I am your father. Such counterpoise challenges particularly the notion of role modeling that valorizes references to mostly dead White men while relegating women and colonized groups to the status of spectacles and never spectators or worse yet actors. Consequently, it is believed that the only kinds of truths a spectacle can produce are the kinds that are good enough only for other spectacles, because original truths, which are considered the universal truths, can be produced only by spectators and their actors. Truth, like common sense, is not common or universal - it is relative and must be understood and interrogated within the politics, time, and space of particular locations.

Health promotion and disease prevention programs designed for African countries should foreground African philosophy, its cultural codes, values, and practices, in order to authenticate relevance in program outcome. This book echoes what has long been recognized - that is, any attempt to provide health solutions for a given community or society must take into serious consideration cultural factors as well as the present stage of the transformation of the society. Thus, the degree to which new programs are co-created to be sustainable is dependent on the extent to which they are culturally appropriate. Program planners and implementers should ensure that the method of health communication is in accord with the cultural reality, consistent with the society's pattern of knowledge acquisition. For this to occur, the health promoters must understand, learn, and develop the skills they will need to reflect appropriately the cultural values of the target population. Doing this requires an understanding not only of the cultural significance of health behaviors but also of the interplay between culture and power relative to policy formulations and decision making at the multilayered levels of a society and its government.

A major aspect of this process entails an understanding of how people promote and/or challenge policies that affect them within their cultural codes and meanings. In other words, one cannot assume that people are disempowered to make decisions based on their economically disadvantaged location. Women and other marginalized groups have always devised passive resistance strategies to subvert oppression. This point can be illustrated by the story of the wise bird. There was once a man who found a beautiful bird, fell in love with it, and decided that he wanted it for a pet. He captured the bird, brought it home, and kept it in a cage. After some days, the man asked the bird if there was anything he could do for the bird. "Of course," the bird responded, "you can open this cage." "I am sorry I cannot do that," said the man, 'but I can take a message to your family to let them know that you are in good health." The bird agreed, and off the man went to find the bird's family. He successfully located the family and delivered the message of the bird's good health and safety. Upon hearing the news, one of the bird's brothers fell dead. The man was shocked at what had happened and could not wait to get home to relate the sad event to "his" bird. Upon hearing the news about his brother, and to the man's surprise, the bird the man had imprisoned also dropped dead. The man, now filled with sorrow, opened the cage, and the bird quickly got up and flew out. As he flew away, he sang to the man, "Thank you for bringing me the wisdom of my people."

The collective experience of a people (the culture) prepares them to deal with and sometimes subvert and transform oppressive conditions in ways unknown to the oppressor. Such experiences and their resultant wisdom transcend levels of income, age, and generation. We must never assume that because a group is economically poor its members are also cerebrally, philosophically, and culturally poor, nor should we assume that wisdom in and of itself will overcome economic oppression. Programmatic efforts must, therefore, be directed toward synchronizing the philosophy of the people with their practices. According to Ngugi Thiong'O (1993), what is needed is a philosophy of practice rather than practical philosophy. We must transform the propagation of binary opposition between the local and the universal, particularly as it relates to culture rather than universalist dogma, which postulates that cultures within a nation and between nations have developed on parallel lines toward parallel ends that never meet.

The challenge for professionals in health and education is to learn to interrogate their relatively privileged position before adopting any strategy for improving health conditions. Empowerment of and participation by the people a program is intended to benefit must consider the degree to which individual decisions are mediated by power, politics, class, and cultural understanding of the meaning of participation and empowerment. Empowerment must be interrogated to address the heightened sense of anxiety that may result from raising individuals' consciousness without also supplying them with the skills, power, and knowledge they need to engage the kinds of emancipatory decisions their new awareness encourages. To engage in a healthy culture project is to question one's location constantly, always remembering that when something stands, another thing always stands beside it.

NOW:

Affirming Our Cultural Wealth

The original impetus for writing about culture and health was to make visible that "other thing" Achebe declared ought to stand beside the "one thing", to bring into the light that which has long been consigned to the shadows. The reflections of my sixteen kindred cultural scholars/workers have done just that, erasing the shadow by illuminating our cultural wealth far more brilliantly than I alone could have achieved. For this, I am deeply grateful for their generosity of cultural and spiritual gifts. They have brought to life the meaning of cultural healing, particularly African culture and, by extension, Global South spaces and lived experiences. In my view, it is not enough simply to make culture visible. We must go beyond what I have called cultural strength, a counterpoint to the popular notion of cultural barrier, to articulate, elevate, and affirm cultural wealth.

In the introduction, I wrote that the very tool we use to express our thoughts and soul, language, is one we are still learning to improve. Much of the Western paradigm elevates its physical and social experiences above others. Well-being is defined largely by physical health and material wealth. In public health, it is widely accepted that wealth (assets over liabilities) is a better predictor of health status than socio-economic measures like employment and income. Yet wealth is almost always understood in purely economic terms.

This thirtieth-year edition is as much about decolonizing the language that contrasts "the West and the rest" as it is about re-imagining new ways of speaking about cultural honors and values, those too often treated as incidental to human experience, by elevating them to their rightful status as ***Cultural Wealth***. I define cultural wealth as the collective honors, values, and ways of being and knowing that sustain, nurture, and elevate a group's sense of identity and connectedness. The practices that embody this connectedness carry invisible emotional and social health benefits that cannot be fully experienced outside their cultural contexts. One example is the honoring of seniority and elderhood through respectful greetings that are central to Nigerian cultures. The common thread running through the interviews that make up the *Now* of this edition is precisely this invisible cultural wealth. Together, the contributors' voices affirm the richness of culture on its own terms, without seeking validation through comparison with the Western paradigm.

In July 2025, I spent most of the month in Nigeria, splitting my time between family in Benin City, my hometown, and projects in Lagos and Abuja. In each city, I was reminded of my own cultural wealth through the way I was welcomed and greeted at every encounter. This began the moment I arrived at Lagos airport. From deplaning to passing through passport control, I must have walked past more than two dozen airport staff, each one welcoming me with our cultural courtesy. This practice of acknowledging and honoring one another with reverence, shared by many African and Asian cultures, is a form of cultural wealth we often take for granted. For me, it was not so much the reverence, often a bow, shown to my personhood as one who is considered an elder, but also my being quickly reminded of the value of reciprocating their reverence with a response of gratitude for being so honored and visibly affirmed. Living in the US meant that I needed such a reminder each time I found myself in spaces that affirmed my cultural wealth.

Throughout my time in Benin City, Lagos, and Abuja, I was met with respect, humility, and honor from both young and old. Perhaps because of timing and age, I found myself treasuring these honoring gestures more deeply than I once did. Their significance became even more striking upon my return to the United States. Back in Atlanta, I felt my cultural wealth being disinvested almost immediately, beginning with the flattening of my seniority into the casual use of my first name by an otherwise friendly Uber driver. The contrast between the affirmation of my elderhood in Nigeria and the reduction to an unseen individual in the U.S. grew sharper when I stepped into the elevator of my building. Three younger people entered, made no eye contact, and offered no greeting. In that moment, the enveloping cultural wealth of honor and reverence I had experienced in three weeks in Nigeria dissipated. The silent entrance and departure of these young, harmless individuals introduced weighty deficits into my otherwise rich cultural experience. It reminded me of the richness of culture that is often invisible in societies where individual physical and material acquisitions are the only values that seem to matter.

We are living in politically disruptive times that affect how we do public health work. In this moment, I can't help but recall my 2007 book *Healing Our Differences: The Politics of Global Health and the Crisis of Identity*. The crisis of identity really does capture today's political and social reality. Efforts to affirm the place of diversity, inclusion, and equity have become a new battleground. As we train the next generation, our focus must be on centralizing cultural wealth and the social structures, systems, and institutions that sustain and celebrate them. This was the central lesson I gained from the sixteen kindred scholars/workers whose reflections gave voice to the *Now* of this edition. The work of elevating and visibilizing cultural strength and wealth will continue in my next book, where I will further illuminate these ideas as part of my own cultural journey, which I have named *My Forward Star*.

I will close as I did in the introduction to the 1995 edition of Health and Culture. This new edition, like the original, seeks to reinscribe culture at the core of public health, health promotion/education, communication, development, and other spaces committed to promoting positive health behavior. It does so in a way that centers the voices of the unheard, the oppressed, and the marginalized in framing and transforming their collective identities. Such a transformative process reinforces the message this book championed more than three decades ago: the time to go beyond the Western paradigm is 'NOW.'

References

THEN AND NOW:

1. Achebe, C. (1987). *Anthills of the savannah*. Garden City, NY: Anchor/Doubleday.

2. Achebe, C. (1992). Interviews with writers of the Post-Colonial World. Edited by Feroza Jussawalla & Reed Way Dasenbrock, Jackson & London: University Press of Mississippi.

3. Ademuwagun, Z. A. (1974-1975). The meeting point of orthodox health personnel and traditional healers/midwives in Nigeria: The pattern of utilization of health services in Ibarapa Division. *Rural Africana*, 26, 55-78.

4. Airhihenbuwa, C. O. (1987). Nigerian heads of households' attitude toward modern and traditional medicines. *Journal of Rural Health*, 3 (11), 21-30.

5. Airhihenbuwa, C. O. (1989a). Health education for African Americans: A neglected task. *Health Education*, 20 (5), 9-14.

6. Airhihenbuwa, C. O. (1989b). Perspectives on AIDS in Africa: Strategies for prevention and control. *AIDS Education and Prevention*, 1, 57-69.

7. Airhihenbuwa, C. O. (1990-1991). A conceptual model for culturally appropriate health education programs in developing countries. *International Quarterly of Community Health Education*, 11(1), 53-62.

8. Airhihenbuwa, C. O. (1992). Health promotion and disease prevention strategies for African-Americans. In R. L. Braithwaite & S. E. Taylor (Eds.), *Health issues in the Black community* (pp.267-280). San Francisco: Jossey-Bass.

9. Airhihenbuwa, C. O. (1993). Health promotion for child survival in Africa: Implications for cultural appropriateness. *International Journal of Health Education*, 12(3), 10-15.

10. Airhihenbuwa, C. O., DiClemente, R. J., Wingood, G. M., & Lowe, A. (1992). HIV/ AIDS education and prevention among African-Americans: A focus on culture. *AIDS Education and Prevention*, 4, 267-276.

11. Airhihenbuwa, C. O., & Lowe, A. G. (1994). Improving the health status of African-Americans: Empowerment as health education intervention. In I. L. Livingston (Ed.), *Handbook of Black American health: The mosaic of conditions, issues, policies and prospects* (pp. 387-398). Westport, CT: Greenwood Press.

12. Airhihenbuwa, C. O., Olsen, L. K., St. Pierre, R. W., & Wang, M. Q. (1989). Race and gender: An analysis of the granting of doctoral degrees in health education programs. *Health Education*, 20(3), 4-7.

13. Airhihenbuwa, C. O., & Pineiro, O. (1988). Cross-cultural health education: A pedagogical challenge. *Journal of School Health*, 58, 240-242.

14. Airhihenbuwa CO. (2007) 2007 SOPHE Presidential Address: On Being Comfortable With Being Uncomfortable: Centering an Africanist Vision in Our Gateway to Global Health. *Health Educ Behav*. 34(1):31-42. doi:10.1177/1090198106291377

15. Airhihenbuwa, C. O. & Iwelunmor eds (2022) Health, Culture and Place: From the Tree to the Forest, U-RISE.org. Atlanta. GA

16. Airhihenbuwa CO (2007) Healing Our Differences: The Crisis of Global Health and the Politics of Identity. Roman and Littlefield. Lanham, Maryland

17. Airhihenbuwa, C. O., Ford, C., Iwelunmor, J., Griffith, D. M., Ameen, K., Murray, T., & Nwaozuru, U. (2024). Decolonization and antiracism: intersecting pathways to global health equity. Ethnicity & Health, 29(7), 846-860.

18. Akerele, O. (1984). WHO's Traditional Medicine Programme: Progress and perspectives. *WHO Chronicle*, 38(2), 76-81.

19. Akerele, O. (1986). The best of both worlds. *Social Science and Medicine*, 21, 177-181.

20. Akinjogbin, I. A. (1990). Reflections on the Nigerian experience. In UNESCO, *Tradition and development in Africa today*. Paris: UNESCO. (Original work published 1987)

21. Alcoff, L. (1991-1992). The problem of speaking for others. *Cultural Critique*, 17, 5-32.

22. Aldous, J. (1969). Wives' employment status and lower-class men as husband-fathers: Support for the Moynihan thesis. *Journal of Marriage and the Family*, 31, 469-476.

23. Allen, R. L. (2004) Whiteness and Critical Pedagogy, Educational Philosophy and Theory, 36(2), 121-136.

24. Allen, R. L. & Rossatto, C. A. (2009). Does Critical Pedagogy Work with Privileged Students? Teacher Education Quarterly, 36(1), pp. 163-180

25. Allen, W. (1978). The search for applicable theories of Black family life. *Journal of Marriage and the Family*, 40, 117-129.

26. American Public Health Association, Governing Council. (1974). *APHA Policy Statement 7424: Racism in the health care delivery system.* Washington, DC: Author.

27. Amos, V., & Parmar, P. (1984). Challenging imperial feminism. *Feminist Review*, 17, 7-19.

28. Anderson, C. A. (1966). Literacy and schooling on the development threshold: Some historic cases. In C. A. Anderson & M. Bowman (Eds.), *Education and economic development.* London: Frank Cass.

29. Asante, M. K. (1983). *Afrocentricity.* Trenton, NJ: African World Press.

30. Asante, M. K. (1987). *The Afrocentric idea.* Philadelphia: Temple University Press.

31. Auslander, W. F., Haire-Joshu, D., Houston, C. A., & Fisher, E. B. (1992). Community organization to reduce the risk of non-insulin-dependent diabetes among low-income African-American women. *Ethnicity and Disease*, 2, 176-184.

32. Baldwin, J. (1981). Notes on an Afrocentric theory of Black personality testing. *Western Journal of Black Studies*, 5(3), 172-179.

33. Bandura, A. (1977). Self-efficacy: Toward a unifying theory of behavioral change. *Psychological Review*, 84, 191-215.

34. Bannerman, R. H., Burton, J., & Wen-Chieh, C. (1983). *Traditional medicine and health care coverage: A reader for health administrators and practitioners*. Geneva: World Health Organization.

35. Basch, P. F. (1990). *International health*. New York: Oxford University Press.

36. Becker, M. H. (1986). The tyranny of health promotion. *Public Health Review*, 14, 15-25.

37. Bell, D. (1992). *Faces at the bottom of the well: The permanence of racism*. New York: Basic Books.

38. Bell, N. K. (1989). AIDS and women: Remaining ethical issues. *AIDS Education and Prevention*, 1, 22-30.

39. Biasio, L. R. (2016). Vaccine hesitancy and health literacy. *Human Vaccines & Immunotherapeutics*, v *13*(3), 701–702. https://doi.org/10.1080/21645515.2016.1243633

40. Bradford, A. S. & Morales, A. E. (2021): Toward a Critical Latinx Pedagogy: A Multi- Generational Reflection on Teaching and Learning in the U.S. Latinx History Survey and Beyond, Journal of Latinos and Education.

41. Braithwaite, R. L., & Lythcott, N. (1989). Community empowerment as a strategy for health promotion for Black and other minority populations. *Journal of the American Medical Association*, 261, 282-283.

42. Burger, M. & Delaloye, L. 2016. The framing of argumentation in the making of a political editorial: From normative expectations to individual credo of the journalists. *Journal of Argumentation in Context* 5(1) 29–47. DOI: 10.1075/jaic.5.1.02bur issn 2211–4742

43. Charatz-Litt, C. (1992). A chronicle of racism: The effects of the White medical community on Black health. *Journal of the National Medical Association*, 84, 717-725.

44. Chinweizu, & Jemie, O. (1987). *Decolonizing the African mind.* London: Sundoor.

45. Chinweizu, Jemie, O., & Madubuike, I. (1983). *Toward the decolonization of African literature: Vol. 1. African fiction and poetry and their critics.* Washington, DC: Howard University Press.

46. Chow, R. (1991). *Women and Chinese modernity: The politics of reading between West and East.* Minneapolis: University of Minnesota Press.

47. Christian, B. (1987). The race for theory. *Cultural Critique*, 6, 52.

48. Cochran, S. D. (1990). Women and HIV infection: Issues in prevention and behavior change. In V. M. Mays, G. W. Albee, & S. F. Schneider (Eds.), *Primary prevention of AIDS: Psychological approaches.* Newbury Park, CA: Sage.

49. Collison, M. N. K. (1992, September 30). Network of Black students hopes to create a new generation of civil rights leaders. *Chronicle of Higher Education*, pp.A28-A29.

50. Davidson, J. M. (1982). Physician participation in Medicaid: Background and issues. *Journal of Health Politics and Policy Law*, 6, 703.

51. Davis, A. Y. (1992). Black nationalism: The sixties and the nineties. In G. Dent (Ed.), *Black popular culture: A project by Michelle Wallace* (pp. 317-324). Seattle: Bay.

52. Davis, G. L., & Cross, H. J. (1979). Sexual stereotyping of Black males in inter-racial sex. *Archives of Sexual Behavior*, 8, 269-279.

53. Davis, J. N. P. (1959). The development of scientific medicine in the African kingdom of Bunga-kitara. *Medical History*, 3(49), 47.

54. Dawit, S., & Mekuria, S. (1993, December 7). The West just doesn't get it. *New York Times*, p.A27.

55. Dennis, R. E. (1985). Health beliefs and practices of ethnic and religious groups. In Watkins & Johnson (Eds.), *Removing cultural and ethnic barriers to health care*. Chapel Hill: University of North Carolina Press.

56. Desmond, S. M., Price, J. H., Hallinan, C., & Smith, D. (1989). Black and White perceptions of their weight. *Journal of School Health*, 59, 353-358.

57. Diop, C. A. (1991). *Civilization or barbarism: An authentic anthropology*. New York: Lawrence Hill.

58. Doyle, E., Smith, C. A., & Hosokawa, M. C. (1989). A process evaluation of a community-based health promotion program for a minority target population. *Health Education*, 20(5), 61-64.

59. Dutta, M. J. (2010). The critical cultural turn in health communication: Reflexivity, solidarity, and praxis. Health communication, 25(6-7), 534-539.

60. Edelman, M. R. (1989). Black children in America. In J. Dewart (Ed.), *The state of Black America 1989* (pp. 63-76). New York: National Urban League.

61. Ellsworth, E. (1989). Why doesn't this feel empowering? Working through the repressive myths of critical pedagogy. Harvard Educational Review, 59(3), p. 297-324.

62. Esteva, G. (1992). Development. In W. Sachs (Ed.), *The development dictionary: A guide to knowledge and power* (pp.6-25). London: Zed.

63. Fanon, F. (1968). *The wretched of the earth.* New York: Grove.

64. Faseke, M. M. (1990). Oral history in Nigeria: Issues, problems, and prospects. *Oral History Review*, 18(1), 77-91.

65. Fingerhut, L. A., & Makuc, D. M. (1992). News from NCHS. *American Journal of Public Health*, 82, 1168-1170.

66. Fishbein, M., & Ajzen, I. (1975). *Belief, attitude, intention, and behavior: An introduction to theory and research.* Reading, MA: Addison-Wesley.

67. Fisher, J. D. (1988). Possible effects of reference group-based social influence on AIDS-risk behavior and AIDS prevention. *American Psychologist*, 43, 914-920.

68. Ford, C. L., & Airhihenbuwa, C. O. (2018). Commentary: just what is critical race theory and what's it doing in a progressive field like public health?. *Ethnicity & disease*, 28(Suppl 1), 223.

69. Ford, C. & Airhihenbuwa, C.O. (2010). Critical Race Theory, Race Equity and Public Health: Toward Antiracism Praxis. *Am J. Public Health,* 100(Suppl 1), S30-S35. doi: 10.2105/AJPH.2009.171058

70. Ford, C. L., Griffith, D. M., Bruce, M. A., & Gilbert, K. L. (Eds.). (2019). *Racism: Science & tools for the public health professional*. American Public Health Association.

71. Foster, E. V. (1963). *Treatment of African mental patients*. Paper presented at the Pan African Psychiatry Conference, Abeokuta, Nigeria.

72. Freire, P. (1970). *Pedagogy of the oppressed*. New York: Continuum.

73. Freire, P. (1973). *Education for critical consciousness*. New York: Continuum.

74. Freire, P. (1993). *Pedagogy of the city*. New York: Continuum.

75. Freire, P., & Faundez, A. (1989). *Learning to question*. New York: Continuum.

76. Fuglesang, A. (1973). *Applied communication in developing countries: Ideas and observations*. New York: Dag Hammarskjld Foundation.

77. Fullilove, M., Fullilove, R. E., Haynes, K. K., & Gross, S. (1990). Black women and AIDS prevention: A view

toward understanding the gender rules. *Journal of Sex Research*, 27(1), 47-64.

78. Gay, G. (2002). Preparing for Culturally Responsive Teaching. Journal of Teacher Education, 53(2), 106-116.

79. Gibson, C. H. (1991). A concept analysis of empowerment. *Journal of Advanced Nursing*, 16, 354-361.

80. Giroux, H. A. (1992). *Border crossings: Cultural workers and the politics of education*. New York: Routledge.

81. Giroux, H. A. (1994a). *Disturbing pleasures: Learning popular culture*. New York: Routledge.

82. Giroux, H. A. (1994b). Living dangerously: Identity politics and the new cultural racism. In H. A. Giroux & P. McLaren (Eds.), *Between borders: Pedagogy and the politics of cultural studies* (pp.29-55). New York: Routledge.

83. Green, E. C. (1988). Can collaborative programs between biomedical and African indigenous health practitioners succeed? *Social Science and Medicine*, 27, 1125-1130.

84. Green, L. W., & Kreuter, M. W. (1991). *Health promotion planning: An educational and environmental approach* (2nd ed.). Palo Alto, CA: Mayfield.

85. Griffiths, W., & Knutson, A. L. (1960). The role of mass media in public health. *American Journal of Public Health*, 50, 515-523.

86. Griffith, D.M., Mason, M., Yonas, M., Eng, E., Jeffries, V., Plihcik, S., & Parks, B. (2007). Dismantling

Institutional Racism: Theory and Action. *American Journal of Community Psychology*, *39*(3-4), 381-392.

87. Gronemeyer, M. (1992). Helping. In W. Sachs (Ed.), *The development dictionary: A guide to knowledge and power* (pp.53-69). London: Zed.

88. Grossberg, L. (1994). Introduction: Bringin' it all back home - pedagogy and cultural studies. In H. A. Giroux & P. McLaren (Eds.), *Between borders: Pedagogy and the politics of cultural studies* (pp. 1-25). New York: Routledge.

89. Gutierrez, L. M. (1990). Working with women of color: An empowerment perspective. *Social Work*, 35, 149-153.

90. Hacker, A. (1992). *Two nations: Black and White, separate, hostile, unequal.* New York: Ballantine.

91. Hale, C. B. (1992). A demographic profile of African Americans. In R. L. Braithwaite & S. E. Taylor (Eds.), *Health issues in the Black community* (pp.6-19). San Francisco: Jossey-Bass.

92. Hall, E. T. (1977). *Beyond culture.* Garden City, NY: Anchor.

93. Hall, S. (1991). Ethnicity: Identity and difference. *Radical America*, 23(4), 9-20.

94. Hall, S. (1992). What is this "Black" in Black popular culture? In G. Dent (Ed.), *Black popular culture: A project by Michelle Wallace* (pp. 21-33). Seattle: Bay.

95. Hall, S., & Jacques, M. (1989). *New times: The changing face of politics in the 1990s.* London: Verso.

96. Hankins, C. A. (1990). Issues involving women, children, and AIDS primarily in the developed world. *Journal of Acquired Immune Deficiency Syndrome*, 3, 443-448.

97. Harrison, I. E. (1974). First International Symposium on Traditional Medical Therapy. *Medical Anthropology Newsletter*, 6(1), 10-13.

98. Harrison, I. E. (1984). *Colonialism, mealth (metropolitan health care) care systems, and traditional healers* (Occasional Paper No. 5). Urbana, IL: Association of Black Anthropologists.

99. Harrison, I. E., & Cosminsky, S. (1976). *Traditional medicine: Implications for ethnomedicine, ethnopharmacology, maternal and child health, mental health, and public health - an annotated bibliography of Africa, Latin America, and the Caribbean.* New York: Garland.

100. Harvey, W. B. (1988). Voodoo and Santeria: Traditional healing techniques in Haiti and Cuba. In C. I. Zeichner (Ed.), *Modern and traditional health care in developing societies: Conflict and cooperation.* New York: University Press of America.

101. Health trends: New vital statistics confirm worsening of Black health. (1992). *Ethnicity and Disease*, 2, 192-193.

102. Holzer, H. (1973). *Beyond medicine.* Chicago: Henry Regnery.

103. hooks, b. (1992). *Black looks: Race and representation.* Boston: South End.

104. hooks, b. (1993, September-October). Let's get real about feminism: The backlash, the myths, the movement. *Ms.*, 4, 34-43.

105. hooks, b. (1994). Teaching to Transgress: Education as the practice of freedom.

106. Hornik, R. (1988). *What are we learning from the evaluation of the Communication for Child Survival project?* Philadelphia: University of Pennsylvania, Annenberg School for Communication, Center for International Health and Development Communication.

107. Horton, E. P., & Smith, J. C. (Eds.). (1990). *Statistical record of Black America.* Detroit: Gale Research.

108. Houston, D. (2015). Red land, living pedagogies: reanimating critical pedagogy through American Indian land justice: response 2. In Red pedagogy: Native American social and political thought (pp. 129-135). Rowman & Littlefield.

109. Illich, I. (1976). *Medical nemesis: The expropriation of health.* New York: Pantheon.

110. Illich, I. (1992). Needs. In W. Sachs (Ed.), *The development dictionary: A guide to knowledge as power* (pp.88-101). London: Zed.

111. International Union of Health Promotion and Education, World Health Organization, & U.S. Centers for Disease Control. (1991). *Meeting global health challenges: A position paper on health education.* Atlanta:

112. Irvine, J. J. (1990). *Black students and school failure: Policies, practices, and prescriptions.* Westport, CT: Greenwood Press.

113. Iwelunmor J, Newsome V, Airhihenbuwa CO. (2014) Framing the impact of culture on health: a systematic review of the PEN-3 cultural model and its application in public health research and interventions. *Ethnicity & Health.* 19(1):20-46. doi:10.1080/13557858.2013.857768

114. Iwelunmor J, Turker JD, Ezechi O, Nwaozuru U, Obiezu-Umeh C, Gbaja-Biamila T, Oladele D, Musa AZ, Airhihenbuwa CO (2023) Sustaining HIV Research in Resource-Limited Settings Using PLAN (People, Leaning, Adapting, Nurturing): Evidence from 4 Youth by Youth Project in Nigeria. *Current HIV AIDS Reports* 20: 111-120.

115. Iwelunmor J, Idris O, Adelakun A, & Airhihenbuwa CO. (2010). Child malaria treatment decisions by mothers of children less than five attending an outpatient clinic in south-west Nigeria: an application of the PEN-3 cultural model. *Malaria Journal,* 9(354).

116. Iwelunmor J; Zungu M; Airhihenbuwa CO. (2010). Rethinking HIV/AID disclosure among women within the context of Motherhood in South Africa, *Am. J. Public Health,* 100(8), 1393-1399.

117. Iwelunmor J. Blackstone S., Vieira D., Nwaozuru U., Airhihenbuwa C, Munodawafa D, Kalipeni E, Jutal A, Shelley D, Ogedegebe, G. (2016). Toward sustainability of health interventions in sub-Saharan Africa: A systematic review. *Implementation Science,* 11(43), 1-27.

118. Jaccard, J., Turrisi, R., & Wan, C. K. (1990). Implications of behavioral decision theory and social marketing for designing social action programs. In J. Edwards, R.20S. Tindale, L. Heath, & C. J. Posavac (Eds.), *Social influence processes and prevention*. New York: Plenum.

119. Jackson, A. M. (1983a). The Black patient and traditional psychotherapy: Implications and possible extensions. *Journal of Community Psychology*, 11, 303-307.

120. Jackson, A. M. (1983b). A theoretical model for the practice of psychotherapy with Black populations. *Journal of Black Psychology*, 10(1), 19-27.

121. Jacob, J. E. (1989). Black America, 1988: An overview. In J. Dewart (Ed.), *The state of Black America 1989* (pp. 1-7). New York: National Urban League.

122. Janzen, J. M. (1974-1975). Pluralistic legitimization of therapy systems in contemporary Zaire. *Rural Africana*, 26, 105-122.

123. Jiménez, K. P. (2006). "Start with the land": Groundwork for Chicana Pedagogy. In D. D. Bernal, C. A. Elenes, F. E. Godinez, & S. Villenas (Eds.), Chicana/Latinx education in everyday life: Femenista perspectives on pedagogy and epistemology. State University of New York.

124. Jones, J. (1982). *Bad blood: The Tuskegee syphilis experiment - a tragedy of race and medicine*. New York: Free Press.

125. Jordan, B. (1989). Cosmopolitan obstetrics: Some insights from the training of traditional midwives. *Social Science and Medicine*, 28, 925-944.

126. Justice, J. (1987). The bureaucratic context of international health: A social scientist's view. *Social Science and Medicine*, 25, 1301-1306.

127. Kaufman-Kurzrock, R. D. (1989). Cultural aspects of nutrition. *Topics in Clinical Nutrition*, 4(2), 1-6.

128. Keeling, R. (1992, April). *Taking the next steps in HIV prevention in young adults*. Paper presented at the Sixth International Conference on AIDS Education, Arlington, VA.

129. Kegley, C. F., & Saviers, A. N. (1983). Working with others who are not like me. *Journal of School Health*, 53(2), 81-85.

130. Kieffer, C. H. (1984). Citizen empowerment: A developmental perspective. In J. Rappaport, C. Swift, & R. Hess (Eds.), *Studies in empowerment: Steps toward understanding and action* (pp.9-36). New York: Haworth.

131. Kisekka, M. N., & Otesanya, B. N. (1990). *Sexually transmitted disease as a gender issue: Examples from Nigeria and Uganda*. Unpublished manuscript.

132. Kreuter, M. W. (1992). PATCH: Its origin, basic concepts and links to contemporary public health policy. *Journal of Health Education*, 23(3), 135-139.

133. Kumanyika, S. K., & Golden, P. M. (1991). Cross-sectional differences in health status in U.S. racial/ethnic minority groups: Potential influence of temporal

changes, disease, and life-style transitions. *Ethnicity and Disease*, 1, 50-59.

134. Kumanyika, S. K., Wilson, J. F., & Guilford-Davenport, M. (1993). Weight-related attitudes and behaviors of Black women. *Journal of the American Dietetic Association*, 93, 416-422.

135. Ladson-Billings, G. (1997). I know why this doesn't feel empowering: A critical "race" analysis of critical pedagogy. Mentoring the Mentor: A Critical Dialogue with Paulo Freire, 60, p. 127-141.

136. Ladson-Billings, G. (2014). Culturally relevant pedagogy 2.0: a.k.a. the Remix. Harvard Educational Review, 84(1), 74-84.

137. Lamarine, R. J. (1989). First do no harm. *Health Education*, 20(4), 22-24.

138. Lambo, T. A. (1961). Mental health in Nigeria: Research and technical problems. *World Mental Health*, 13.

139. Lambo, T. A. (1978). Psychotherapy in Africa. *Human Nature*, 1(3), 32-39.

140. Last, M. (1986). The professionalization of African medicine: Ambiguities and definitions. In M. Last & G. L. Chavunduka (Eds.), *The professionalization of traditional medicine*. Manchester, UK: Manchester University Press/International African Institute.

141. Lau, R. R., Quadrel, M. J., & Hartman, K. A. (1990). Development and change of young adults' preventive health beliefs and behavior: Influence of parents and

peers. *Journal of Health and Social Behavior*, 31, 240-259.

142. Leonard, P., & Jones, A. C. (1980). Theoretical considerations for psychotherapy with Black clients. In R. C. Jones (Ed.), *Black psychology* (2nd ed.). New York: Harper & Row.

143. Levy, D. R. (1985). White doctors and Black patients: Influence of race on the doctor-patient relationship. *Pediatrics*, 75, 639-643.

144. Lewin, K. (1947). Group decision and social change. In A. Swanson, T. M. Newcomb, & Z. L. Hartley (Eds.), *Readings in social psychology* (pp.197-211). Englewood Cliffs, NJ: Prentice Hall.

145. Lynn, M., Jennings, M. E. & Hughes, S. (2013) Critical race pedagogy 2.0: lessons from Derrick Bell, Race Ethnicity and Education, 16(4), 603-628.

146. Maclean, L. M., & Bannerman, R. H. (1982). Utilization of indigenous healers in national health delivery systems. *Social Science and Medicine*, 16, 1815-1816.

147. Malinowski, B. (1954). The rationalization of anthropology and administration. *Africa*, 3, 405-429.

148. Marable, M. (1993). Beyond racial identity politics: Towards a liberation theory for multicultural democracy. *Race and Class*, 35(1), 113-130.

149. Mariani, P., & Crary, J. (1990). In the shadow of the West: An interview with Edward Said. In R. Ferguson, W. Olander, M. Turker, & K. Fiss (Eds.), *Discourses: Conversations in postmodern art and culture*. New

York/Cambridge: New York Museum of Contemporary Art/MIT Press.

150. Mays, V. M., & Cochran, S. D. (1988). Issues in the perception of AIDS risk and risk reduction activities by Black and Latino women. *American Psychologist*, 43, 949-957.

151. Mazrui, A. A. (1986). *The Africans: A triple heritage*. Boston: Little, Brown.

152. McCarty, T. L. & Lee, T. S. (2014). Critical culturally sustaining/revitalizing pedagogy and Indigenous education sovereignty. Harvard Educational Review, 84(1), 101-124.

153. McNair-Knox, F. C. (1991). Tapping into teen talk: Parenting strategies for bridging the intergenerational communication gap. In B. P. Bowser (Ed.), *Black male adolescents: Parenting and education in community context*. New York: University Press of America.

154. McNamara, R. S. (1973, September 24). Address to the Board of Governors, World Bank, Nairobi.

155. Miles, G. B., & McDavis, R. J. (1982). Effects of four orientation approaches on disadvantaged Black freshmen students' attitudes toward the counseling center. *Journal of College Student Personnel*, 23, 413-418.

156. Minh-ha, T. T. (1989). *Woman, nature, other: Writing postcoloniality and feminism*. Bloomington: Indiana University Press.

157. Minh-ha, T. T. (1991). *When the moon waxes red: Representation, gender and cultural politics*. New York: Routledge.

158. Mitchell, J. L. (1988). Women, AIDS, and public policy. *AIDS and Public Policy Journal*, 3(2), 50-52.

159. Mohanty, C. T. (1991a). Introduction: Cartographies of struggle. In C. T. Mohanty, A.20Russo, & L. Torres (Eds.), *Third World women and the politics of feminism* (pp. 1-47). Bloomington: Indiana University Press.

160. Mohanty, C. T. (1991b). Under Western eyes: Feminist scholarship and colonial discourses. In C. T. Mohanty, A. Russo, & L. Torres (Eds.), *Third World women and the politics of feminism* (pp.51-80). Bloomington: Indiana University Press.

161. Morales, E. S. (1987). AIDS and ethnic minority research. *Multicultural Inquiry and Research on AIDS*, 1, 2.

162. Morrison, T. (1992). *Playing in the dark: Whiteness and the literary imagination*. New York: Vintage.

163. Mudimbe, V. Y. (1988). *The invention of Africa: Gnosis, philosophy, and the order of knowledge*. Bloomington: Indiana University Press.

164. Mullen, P. D., Hersey, J. C., & Iverson, D. C. (1987). Health models compared. *Social Science and Medicine*, 24, 973-981.

165. Muller, C. (1985). A window on the past: The position of the client in twentieth century public health thought and practice. *American Journal of Public Health*, 75, 470-476.

166. Myers, H. F., & King, L. M. (1983). Mental health issues in the development of the Black American child.

In G. J. Powell (Ed.), *The psychosocial development of minority group children.* New York: Brunner/Mazel.

167. Nathanson, C. A., & Becker, M. H. (1986). Family and peer influence on obtaining a method of contraception. *Journal of Marriage and the Family*, 48, 513-525.

168. Newman, A., & Bhatia, J. C. (1973). Family planning and indigenous medicine practitioners. *Social Science and Medicine*, 14A, 23-29.

169. Nichols, M. (1990). Women and acquired immunodeficiency syndrome: Issues for prevention. In B. Voeller, J. M. Reinisch, & M. Gottlieb (Eds.), *AIDS and sex: An integrated biomedical and biobehavioral approach.* New York: Oxford University Press.

170. Njoku, J. E. E. (1980). *The world of the African woman.* Metuchen, NJ: Scarecrow.

171. Nobles, W. W. (1980). African philosophy: Foundations for Black psychology. In R. L. Jones (Ed.), *Black psychology* (2nd ed.). New York: Harper & Row.

172. Nobles, W. W. (1985). Back to the roots: African culture as a basis for understanding black families. In W. W. Nobles (Ed.), *Africanity and the Black family: The development of a theoretical model.* Berkeley, CA: Institute for the Advanced Study of Black Family Life and Culture.

173. Nwaozuru U, Ikuomola OB, Obiezu-Umeh C, Shato T. (2022). Mapping the Application of the PEN-3 Cultural Model: Over 30 Years in Play. In Airhihenbuwa

CO and Iwelunmor JI Eds. *Health, Culture and Place: From the Tree to the Forest.* U-RISE. Atlanta, GA

174. Nwaozuru U, Murphy P, Richard A, Obiezu-Umeh C, Shato T, Obionu I, Gbajabiamila T, Oladele D, Mason S, Takenaka BP, Blessing LA, Engelhart A, Nkengasong S, Chinaemerem ID, Anikamadu O, Adeoti E, Patel P, Ojo T, Olusanya O, Shelley D, Airhihenbuwa C, Ogedegbe G, Ezechi O, Iwelunmor J. (2025) The sustainability of health interventions implemented in Africa: an updated systematic review on evidence and future research perspectives. *Implement Sci Commun.* 8;6(1):39. doi: 10.1186/s43058-025-00716-x. PMID: 40200368; PMCID: PMC11980204.

175. Nzegwu N.U. (2006) *Family Matters: Feminist Concepts in African Philosophy of Culture.* Albany, State University of New York.

176. Nzegwu N.U. ed (2014). *Onitsha at the Millennium: Legacy, History and Transformation,* vol 2. Endicott, NY: Africa Resource Press.

177. Obregon R & Waisbord S. (2012) *The Handbook of Global Health Communication.* Wiley-Blackwell.

178. Okoror, T.A. & & Airhihenbuwa, C.O., Shisana, O., Zungu-Dirwayi, N., Smith, E., Brown, D., & Louw J. (2008). “My mother told me I must not cook anymore” - Food, Culture, and the Contexts of HIV and AIDS related Stigma in Three Communities in South Africa. *The International Quarterly for Community Health Education,* 28(3), 201-213.

179. Osuntokun, B. O. (1975). The traditional basis of neuropsychiatric practice among the Yorubas of Nigeria. *Tropical Geographic Medicine*, 27, 422-430.

180. Oyebola, D. D. O. (1986). National medical policies in Nigeria. In M. Last & G. L. Chavunduka (Eds.), *The professionalization of traditional medicine*. Manchester, UK: Manchester University Press/International African Institute.

181. Ozer, E. M., & Bandura, A. (1990). Mechanisms governing empowerment effects: A self-efficacy analysis. *Journal of Personality and Social Psychology*, 58, 472-486.

182. Parham, T. A., & Helms, J. E. (1985). Relation of racial identity attitudes to self-actualization and affective states of Black students. *Journal of Counseling Psychology*, 32, 431-440.

183. Paris, D. (2012). Culturally Sustaining Pedagogy: A Needed Change in Stance, Terminology, and Practice, Educational Researcher, 41(3), 93–97.

184. Parker, S., & Kleiner, R. (1969). Social psychological dimensions of the family role performance of the Negro male. *Journal of Marriage and the Family*, 33, 500-506.

185. Pedersen, P., Draguns, J., Conner, W., & Trimble, J. (1981). *Counseling across cultures*. Honolulu: University of Hawaii Press/East-West Center.

186. Pernick, M. S. (1985). *A calculus of suffering*. New York: Columbia University Press.

187. Petersdorf, P. G., Turner, K. S., Nickens, H. W., & Ready, T. (1990). Minorities and medicine: Past, present, and future. *Academic Medicine*, 65, 663-670.

188. Peterson, J. L., & Bakerman, R. (1989). AIDS and IV drug use among ethnic minorities. *Journal of Drug Issues*, 19(1), 27-37.

189. Pike, K. L. (1954). *Language in relation to a unified theory of the structure of human behavior: Part 1* (preliminary ed.). Summer Institute of Linguistics.

190. Pillsbury, B. L. K. (1982). Policy and evaluation perspectives on traditional health practitioners in national health care systems. *Social Science and Medicine*, 16, 1825-1834.

191. Proctor, E., & Rosen, A. (1981). Expectations and preferences for counselor race and their relation to intermediate treatment outcomes. *Journal of Counseling Psychology*, 28, 40-46.

192. Radcliffe-Brown, A. R. (1952). *Structure and function in primitive society: Essays and addresses*. Glencoe, IL: Free Press.

193. Rahnema, M. (1992). Participation. In W. Sachs (Ed.), *The development dictionary: A guide to knowledge and power* (pp.116-131). London: Zed.

194. Rappaport, J. (1981). In praise of paradox: A social policy of empowerment over prevention. *American Journal of Community Psychology*, 9, 1-25.

195. Rappaport, J. (1984). Studies in empowerment: Introduction to the issue. In J. Rappaport, C. Swift, & R. Hess (Eds.), *Studies in empowerment: Steps toward understanding and action* (pp. 1-7). New York: Haworth.

196. Rendón, L. I. (2009). Sentipensante sensing/thinking pedagogy: Educating for wholeness, social justice, and liberation. Stylus

197. Richards, P. 2016. *How a People's Science Helped End an Epidemic.* Zed Books.

198. Rosenstock, I. M. (1974). Historical origins of the health belief model. *Health Education Monographs,* 2, 328-335.

199. Sachs, W. (1992). Introduction. In W. Sachs (Ed.), *The development dictionary: A guide to knowledge and power* (pp.1-5). London: Zed.

200. Saegert, S. (1989). Unlikely leaders, extreme circumstances: Older Black women building community households. *American Journal of Community Psychology,* 17, 295-316.

201. Said, E. (1990) In the Shadow of the West: An interview with Edward Said by Phil Mariani & Jonathan Crary. *Discourses: Conversations in Postmodern Art and Culture.* Edited by: Russell Ferguson, William Olander, Marcia Turker and Karen Fiss. NYC. Cambridge: The New Museum of Contemporary Art and The MIT Press.

202. Sastry S and Dutta MJ. 2017. Health Communication in the Time of Ebola: A Culture-Centered Interrogation. *Journal of Health Communication.* v 22 (sup1):10-14. doi: 10.1080/10810730.2016.1216205. PMID: 28854138.

203. Savitt, T. L. (1982). The use of Blacks for medical experimentation and demonstration in the Old South. *Journal of Southern History,* 48, 331-335.

204. Schram, R. (1971). *A history of Nigerian health services*. Ibadan, Nigeria: Ibadan University Press.

205. Seidel, G. (1993). The competing discourses of HIV/AIDS in sub-Saharan Africa: Discourses of rights and empowerment vs. discourses of control and exclusion. *Social Science and Medicine*, 36, 175-194.

206. Seijas, H. (1975). An approach to the study of medical aspects of culture. *Current Anthropology*, 14, 344-345.

207. Simons, M. (1989, May 16). Poor nations seeking rewards for contributions to plant species. *New York Times*, p.18.

208. Sprafka, J. M., Burke, G. L., Folsom, A. R., & Hahn, L. P. (1989). Hypercholesteremia prevalence, awareness and treatment in Blacks and Whites: The Minnesota Heart Survey. *Preventive Medicine*, 18, 423-432.

209. Stewart, J. B. (1989). *The state of Black studies: Perspectives from the first NCBS Summer Faculty Institute and implications of the NRC report "A common destiny."* Paper presented at Temple University, Philadelphia.

210. Stewart, J. B. (1992). Reaching for higher ground: Toward an understanding of Black/ Africana studies. *Afrocentric Scholar*, 1(1), 1-63.

211. Street, B. V. (1984). *Literacy in theory and practice*. Cambridge, UK: Cambridge University Press.

212. Sullivan, L. W. (1989). Shattuck lecture: The health care priorities of the Bush administration. *New England Journal of Medicine*, 321, 125-128.

213. Teller, A. (1968). Studies on aspects of traditional medicine. *Lagos Notes and Records*, 2(1), 18.

214. Thiam, A. (1986). *Speak out, Black sisters: Feminism and oppression in Black Africa*. London: Pluto.

215. Thiong'O, N. W. (1986). *Decolonizing the mind: The politics of language in African literature*. London: James Currey/Heinemann.

216. Thiong'O, N. W. (1993). *Moving the center: The struggle for cultural freedoms*. London: James Currey.

217. Tones, K., Tilford, S., & Robinson, Y. K. (1991). *Health education: Effectiveness and efficiency*. London: Chapman & Hall.

218. Torrey, E. F. (1972). What Western psychotherapists can learn from witch doctors. *American Journal of Orthopsychiatry*, 42, 69-76.

219. U.N. Development Programme. (1993). *Human development report*. New York: Oxford University Press.

220. Joint United Nations Programme on HIV/AIDS (UNAIDS). 2009. Communications Framework for HIV/AIDS: A New Direction. UNAIDS. Geneva.

221. U.S. Department of Health and Human Services. (1985). *Report of the Secretary's Task Force on Black and Minority Health* (Vol. 1, exec. summary). Washington, DC: Government Printing Office.

222. U.S. Department of Health and Human Services. (1991). *Health of the United States and prevention profile* (NCHS Publication No. PHS 91-1232). Washington, DC: Government Printing Office.

223. U.S. Surgeon General. (1979). *Healthy people: The surgeon general's report on health promotion and disease prevention.* Washington, DC: Government Printing Office.

224. Waitoller, F. R. & Thorius, K. A. K. (2016) Cross-pollinating culturally sustaining pedagogy and universal design for learning: Toward an inclusive pedagogy that accounts for dis/ability. Harvard Educational Review, 86(3), 366-389.

225. Wasike, B. P 2017. Persuasion in 140 Characters: Testing Issue Framing, Persuasion and Credibility via Twitter and Online News Articles in the Gun Control Debate. *Computers in Human Behavior* 66: 179-190. Available [O]: https://doi.org/10.1016/j.chb.2016.09.037 Accessed: 2017/09/26

226. Werner, D. (1989, June 18-21). *Health for no one by the year 2000: The high cost of placing "national security" before global justice.* Address presented to the 16th Annual International Health Conference of the National Council for International Health, Arlington, VA.

227. West, C. (1990). The new cultural politics of difference. In R. Ferguson, M. Geverr, T.20T. Minh-ha, & C. West (Eds.), *Out there: Marginalization and contemporary cultures* (pp. 19-36). Cambridge: MIT Press.

228. West, C. (1993). *Race matters.* Boston: Beacon.

229. Whitehead, T. (1992). In search of soul food and meaning: Culture, food, and health. In H. A. Baer & Y. Jones (Eds.), *African Americans in the South: Issues*

of race, class, and gender (pp.94-110, 161-178). Athens: University of Georgia Press.

230. World Health Organization. (1989). Memoranda: In vitro screening of traditional medicines for anti-HIV activity: Memorandum for a WHO meeting. *Bulletin of the World Health Organization*, 67, 613-618.

231. Wyatt, G. E., Strayer, R. G., & Lobitz, W. C. (1976). Issues in the treatment of sexual dysfunctioning couples of Afro-American descent. *Psychotherapy*, 13, 44-50.

232. Zuberi, T., & Bonilla-Silva, E. (Eds.). (2008). White logic, white methods: Racism and methodology. Rowman & Littlefield.

NOW - Interview Contributors and Affiliation in Alphabetical Order

Ameen, Khadijah, PhD, MPH

Division of Community Health Sciences, School of Public Health

University of California,

Berkeley, CA

Ford, Chandra L., PhD, MPH, MLIS

Department of Behavioral, Social and Health Education Sciences, Rollins School of Public Health

Department of African American Studies, College of Arts and Sciences

Emory University, Atlanta, GA

Griffith, Derek M., PhD

Department of Family and Community Health, School of Nursing

Department of Medical Ethics and Health Policy, Perelman School of Medicine

University of Pennsylvania, Philadelphia, PA

Iwelunmor, Juliet I., PhD

Light Institute for Global Health and Transformation

Washington University in St. Louis, School of Medicine

Saint Louis, MO

Iwuagwu, Stella, PhD, MS, MPH, RN/M
Sustainable Demonstration Farms Limited (SDFarms)
Abuja, Nigeria

Kingori, Caroline, PHD, MPH
Department of Social and Public Health
College of Health Sciences and Professions
Ohio University, Athens OH

Makinwa, Bunmi, MPA
AUNIQUEI Communication for Leadership
Lagos, Nigeria

Madzinga-Kusena, Priscilla, PhD
Africa CDC
Addis Ababa, Ethiopia

Munodawafa, Davison, EdD
Faculty of Medicine and Health Sciences
Midlands State University
Gweru, Zimbabwe.

Ndiaye, Khadidiatou PhD
Department of Prevention & Community Health
The George Washington University
Washington, DC

Nwaozuru, Ucheoma C., PhD
Department of Implementation Science,
Wake Forest School of Medicine
Winston-Salem, NC

Nzegwu, Nkiru U., PhD
Department of Africana Studies and Global Public Health Program
Binghamton University,
Binghamton, New York

Obregon, Rafael A., PhD
Country Representative
UNICEF Nicaragua

Okoror, Titilayo A., PhD
Department of Africana Studies and Global Public Health Program
Binghamton University,
Binghamton, New York

Sharif, Mienah Z., PhD, MPH
Division of Community Health Sciences, School of Public Health
University of California,
Berkeley, CA

Shine, Randy, MS
Shine Entertainment
Philadelphia, PA

Index

THEN AND NOW:

B

C

I

K

L

M

About the Author

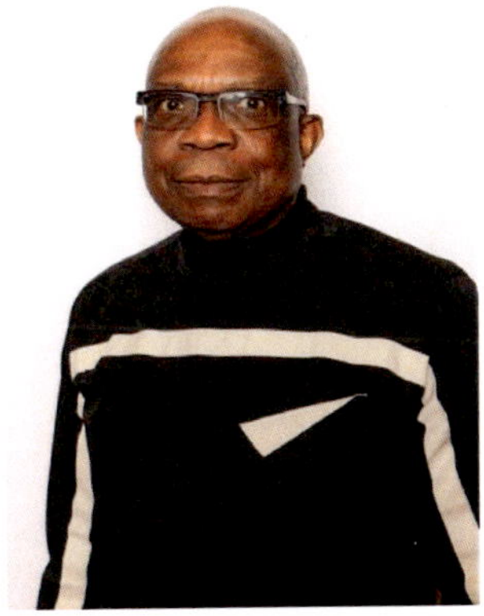

Collins O. Airhihenbuwa is Professor of Global Public Health at Georgia State University and Founding CEO of U-RISE, LLC. A pioneering global health scholar, he is internationally recognized for centralizing culture in global public health. He previously served as Head of the Department of Biobehavioral Health at Penn State University and as Dean of the College for Public Health and Social Justice at Saint Louis University. In 1989, he developed and first published the PEN-3 Model, and in 2010, he co-developed the Public Health Critical Race Praxis with Chandra Ford. Professor Airhihenbuwa has led research collaborations, institutional partnerships, and the mentoring of faculty and professional staff at institutions worldwide. His books include *Health and Culture: Beyond the Western Paradigm* (1995), *Healing Our Differences: The Crisis of Global Health and the Politics of Identity* (2007), and *Health, Culture and Place: From the Tree to the Forest* (2022), co-edited with Juliet Iwelunmor. He remains a tireless leader in centering culture in scholarships and practices to decolonize global public health and advance anti-racism and health equity.

www.ingramcontent.com/pod-product-compliance
Lightning Source LLC
Chambersburg PA
CBRC101212220926
51847CB00006B/55

9789699792243